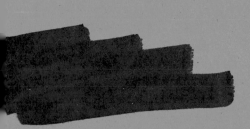

"So You Want to Be a Doctor?"

"So You Want to Be a Doctor?"

THE REALITIES OF PURSUING
MEDICINE AS A CAREER
BY
Naomi Bluestone, M.D.

Lothrop, Lee & Shepard Books
New York

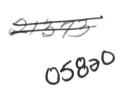

Library of Congress Cataloging in Publication Data
Bluestone, Naomi. "So you want to be a doctor?"
Bibliography: p. 1. Medicine—Vocational guidance—United States. 2. Medical
education—United States. 3. Bluestone, Naomi. 4. Physicians—New York (N.Y.)—
Biography. I. Title.
R690.B63 610'.23'73 81-2545 ISBN 0-688-00739-2 AACR2

For
Simon Alexander Grolnick, M.D.

Acknowledgments

I am indebted to the late Catherine Bryson, who taught me how to write the English language; the late Professor Robert Hillyer, who helped me to appreciate its literature; the late Edith Jacobson, M.D., who encouraged me to use it as a therapeutic tool; and Decia Fates, former editor of *Medical Dimensions*, who gave me the opportunity to implement this excellent advice.

I am also grateful to the many friends, colleagues, students, and correspondents who have gnawed on all kinds of intellectual bones with me through the years and will find fragments of themselves in this volume. Among these I note particularly Drs. David and Ethel Platt.

Finally, I owe a debt of gratitude to my dear father, the late Dr. Harry Bluestone, whose pride in me was very sustaining; my remarkable mother, Miriam Bluestone, who is back in school and writing her memoirs at the age of seventy-three; and, of course, Bob.

Contents

Private Thoughts for Special People

Looking Back and Looking Forward

Getting Started: College

1.
My
Hideous
Example

My cousin Milton, who never let his profession interfere with his enjoyment of the Broadway theater, or the latest C. P. Snow novel, was precisely the kind of doctor who appealed to students considering a career in medicine. He had an avuncular, scholarly look about him, fostered by a well-worn pipe that also managed a hint of his human frailties. It was natural that they should approach him for advice.

"I handle would-be physicians in a very special way," he once said to me, tamping his tobacco deep into its bowl. "First, I congratulate them on having chosen the worthiest and most rewarding of professions. Next, I assure them that I would be proud and happy to have them for colleagues. Then, I tell them everything they can expect. I spare them absolutely nothing. I tell them about the merciless competition, the chronic exhaustion, the ever-present feelings of inadequacy. I tell them that if they don't look sharp, they may never see their families again. I tell them that they will have to master the impossible, live with uncertainty, and break up fecal impactions on an empty stomach. I tell them they will become intellectual slaves, tied hand and foot in red tape, hostages to the agencies that are fueled on malpractice insurance.

3

I remind them that they can get much richer going into business (preferably the malpractice insurance business), and that even if they do make a bundle, their life-styles will not allow them to enjoy it. I lean down hard on the moral and ethical dilemmas in their daily decision making, and the overall costs of bearing the doctor's burden. Believe me, I do everything I possibly can to discourage them."

He took a long, deep puff and smiled his little cat smile. "And then when I've finished raking them over the coals, I walk away and pray to God they won't listen to me and will do it anyway. . . ."

I had every reason to believe that he meant what he said because, although he seemed to have forgotten it, he'd once done the same number on *me*!

When I went off to college, becoming a doctor was the last thing on my mind. I wanted to write the great American novel, and so I majored in English literature. But the first night of my sophomore year, somewhere about 2:00 A.M., I awoke suddenly from sleep with the strange feeling that something wonderful was about to happen. "Wake up, Esther," I said, shaking my roommate out of a well-earned sleep (as she'd been out gamboling and cavorting past midnight). "I'm going to be a *doctor*!" "Go back to sleep," she said. "You're drunk." (I thought that was a pretty classic case of projection, myself, but never mind.)

If I was not drunk, I was clearly in the throes of a sudden emotional and intellectual upheaval, and there was to be no sleep that night. In the morning I went to my faculty adviser and told him that I wanted to go to medical school, and therefore had to switch around all the courses for which I'd just registered the day before. Since I had studiously avoided all elective science courses until that date, he was quite within his rights to suggest that I take my first course at Student Health. But I was not to be dissuaded, and found myself enrolled in elementary physiology, elementary mathematics, and elementary qualitative analysis before the next day was out.

I was not a complete fool, however. Somewhere I'd heard that it wasn't easy being accepted at medical school, and it seemed wise to retain my English major in case I should ever need it. I made it a point to continue my previous college work in addition to the new load, just in case there should be a depression some day and they wouldn't need doctors.

Since in those days I was a pretty docile creature, and craved some validating stamp on my somewhat irregular activities, I thought I'd better run up from the University of Delaware to Brooklyn, New York, on the Pennsylvania Railroad for a whiff of some pipe smoke and a little informed consent from this cousin who was twenty-five years my senior. The entire English department, after all, had been scandalized and hurt at my defection, and who knew what my parents would say when they heard what I had done? Clearly, it was time to talk to Milton. That's when he did his now-familiar number on me.

"So you want to be a doctor!" he proclaimed in his booming voice, which emanated from the middle of four-hundred cubic yards of medical volumes lined up behind him. His phrase reminded me of one of those dumb career books for adolescents: *So you want to be a prima ballerina? So you want to be a collector of Dieffenbachia mutants?* "So you want to be a doctor?" he repeated, the voice filtered through a haze of aromatic smoke. "Wonderful! Marvelous! I'd be proud to have you for a colleague!" Well, *that* was more like it. My grandfather had been a physician, and since most of his sons, sons-in-law, and grandsons had followed the family trade, there were by now twenty or thirty physician-relatives, none of whom, however, was a woman. I was hoping he'd say something like, "How wonderful to have a woman physician among the Bluestone family doctors!" But it was 1955 and something else came out.

"*You're a girl,*" he said. I had been aware of this. "You would have to apply to a school that takes women. There aren't too many."

"I've heard that Penn takes five women out of a hundred and twenty. But there's the Woman's Medical College of Pennsylvania," I gamely replied. "Right," he said, "and my own school, the State University of New York, also has a pretty good record. But you'd have heavy competition." I nodded. Somehow, at that point in my life, the word "competition" didn't have quite the menacing ring it has now.

"*You're a Jew*," he said. That kind of got my hackles up. (Well, at least he didn't call me a *Jewess*!) I was a committed, educated, and knowledgeable Jew, and I *liked* being Jewish. I expected better from my own cousin, who, like it or not, had been born as Jewish as I had been. "Do you remember Uncle Moe's commencement picture, when he graduated from Columbia University's College of Physicians and Surgeons in 1922?" I nodded. "Do you remember all those neat little portraits in ovals, lined up across the page?" I wished he'd get to the point. "Do you know *why* those neat little ovals?" I shook my head slowly from side to side. "Those neat little ovals were because the gentile boys in the class refused to pose for a group photograph with the Jews!"

I was beginning to get the picture. Fortunately, I remembered no *girls* in the class, or their photos might have been printed on the back. What a shame! P and S had always seemed like such a classy, elegant place to me, the perfect place to go to medical school. I was sure it was full of pipe smoke and acres of books with hidden mysteries. Now one thing was certain, there were probably as few Jews as the laws would allow. And experience had taught me that if there were few Jews, there were fewer blacks, no girls, and, I sniffed to myself, probably no one who read C. P. Snow, listened to seventeenth-century chamber music, or believed in the power of beauty to transform. Milton had chalked up another deterrent, and this one was painfully real.

"*You come from a cow college.*" I was really shocked. It was true that most of the serious students at Delaware were engineers who ran around with slide rules sticking out of their hip pockets, thus making the simple act of sitting down a noisy and awkward experience, but the quality of education was superior, and the ivy on our two-hundred-year-old buildings was as green-blooded as that of more famous schools. "It would have helped if you were coming from Vassar or Bryn Mawr." I attempted a lighthearted repartee. "Well, maybe I am a bovine, but I'm not a hayseed; I want to go to medical school, not veterinary school." The humor was lost; another nail was being pounded into my educational coffin because my school was *déclassé*.

"Don't be discouraged," Milton said, his keen diagnostic eye noting the barely discernible sag of my posture. "How are your grades?" I was capable of ruthless honesty, even at the tender age of eighteen. "I got a C in high-school chemistry," I replied. "The teacher didn't like me."

"And your other science courses?" *What* other courses? I wracked my brain. "I took algebra and geometry in high school, and did very poorly, but I don't see what that has to do with medicine. And since I've been at Delaware, I've gotten straight A's in English and allied subjects."

"What about your scientific aptitude tests?" I shrank a bit lower in his wing chair. I could not bring myself to report that the vocational guidance counselor had given high praise to my verbal skills, charitable de-emphasis to my mechanical and quantitative abilities, and had strongly urged that I become a teacher or social worker. The sordid truth of the matter was that I had no scientific aptitude whatsoever, a classic math block, a squeamish stomach, a phobia about arachnids, and so much free-floating anxiety it wasn't even floating any more. "I'll get a tutor if I have to." Milton blanched, and we took a break for tea.

When we reconvened, it was apparent that he had been brooding about my cavalier attitude toward scholastic aptitude. The first thing he did when he returned to his desk was to pull a book at random from his shelves. It had print finer than the Manhattan phone book and was at least as large. Bound in hard cover, it was so heavy I could not handle it without straining both hands and the muscles of my upper arms as well. "Take a long, hard look," he said. "Ask yourself if you have the brains and guts to sit with a book like that, and countless more besides, till all hours of the night, studying, cramming, and knowing that you must master it or someday someone will die unnecessarily because you weren't good enough. Can you stick with it to the end?"

It was truly a dramatic moment, and one I will not forget. The silence hung as heavy as the dead smoke in the air. I honestly don't remember how I replied, but knowing me, it must have been something grandiose and emotional. I was convinced that I would learn that damn textbook of physiology if I had to look up every one of its polysyllabic words in the dictionary . . . and I'd have it memorized by morning.

"I think you should also be considering the costs of a medical education," my mentor resumed a few moments later. "Tuition can run you over a thousand dollars a year, plus your room, board, and supplies. Books alone can be a hefty item." I could well believe that physiology text would not come cheap, and rose to the occasion. "I will have saved up enough for the first year by the time I graduate. After that, I will take a loan." Brave words from a woman whose single major expenditure in the past ten years had been $220 for half a silver flute (the other half supplied by loving parents). "You may have to consult with your father on that," he said smoothly, ominously.

We talked about many other things that day. As I look back on the interview, I realize that Milton had touched only on reality, and environmental, rather than personal, reality at that. He had introduced only those considerations and possible impediments that were certain to cause trouble. He discussed the issues of discrimination, finances, intellectual capability, and capacity to follow a difficult goal to its conclusion. But he had neglected to discuss the many other issues that were to prove equally as threatening. He did not talk too much about having to give up parties, significant family and life events, necessary sleep, fun and recreation. He did not talk about how awful it could be to do animal experimentation, or be plunged into a hospital job without adequate preparation for the painful sights and experiences that are part of such a position. Despite his conviction that he did everything in his power to turn students off, the better to weed out those who could and should pursue other goals, he had gone fairly easy on me. Maybe I was a favorite cousin and so young and eager he hadn't the heart to put his shoe on my face. Maybe he really did think I knew the score and had what it took to overcome the dismal reality. Or maybe he was just feeling mellow that day. But if you think Milton worked me over, consider what happened when I went home the following weekend and announced my plans to my unsuspecting parents. My mother became lyrically hysterical, her voice rising two full octaves above its conversational norm. She was spared an apoplectic attack only by the belief that I couldn't possibly be serious about what I was proposing. Unable to confront me directly, she resorted to referring to me in the impersonal pronoun.

"*This* wants to be a doctor!" she emoted. "*This*, who got a C in high-school chemistry!" (She'd never forgiven me for that.) "*This*, who can't even keep her room clean! *This* wants to be a *doctor*?" It did me no good to hear, as the full import of Milton's warnings had started to sink in, and I was already half in agreement with her. In vain I looked to my father for some reassurance that I was not a complete loon.

"Really, Miriam," he said, "leave the girl alone. If she wants to be a doctor, she should be a doctor! I'm sure she is smart enough to do it, if she puts her mind to it. What I can't understand is *why* she would want to do it!" He, too, seemed to be referring to me as if I weren't there. "Who would want to marry a lady doctor? She'll *never* have a husband, *never* have children, some price she'll pay. But if that's what she wants, what's it to you? And what does keeping her room clean have to do with it? Without a husband, what does it matter if her room is clean or it isn't?" He took his logic to his favorite piece of upholstery and hid behind the Journal-Every-Evening. If he'd smoked a pipe, he surely would have lit it.

My mother realized quickly enough that her tactics had been tangential to the real cause of dissuading me from my folly. She knew a good line when she heard one. "Doesn't it *bother* you that you will never have a husband?" she inquired, accepting this consequence as a "given." "Nonsense," I replied, my ovaries in knots. "Where's a better place to meet men than in a medical school?" "As you wish," she replied, her voice implying that I would not hear the end of it.

My parents' attitude was not difficult to understand, considering that they had been ravaged, like so many others, by the Great Depression. Security was life. My mother had made it clear from my earliest childhood that she thought I would be best off being a teacher. I could come home at four o'clock each day and have time to care for my children and make dinner for my husband. I would have summers off to supplement my earnings as a camp counselor, and get free placement in the country for the kids. In case my husband would ever be out of work or, God forbid, leave me for a tinny blonde, I would be able to support myself. And there would be a pension. I was certainly expected to go to college to become a well-rounded liberal arts major, but aspiring to go to medical school was carrying this accomplishment *schtick* just a little too far.

My father, who was not a physician, believed incontrovertibly in the education of women, as long as it did not interfere with their chances of marital success. To him, the saddest spectacle in this world was an "older girl" who had failed to catch the brass ring on the merry-go-round of life. Not even becoming a physician should jeopardize this goal for his darling younger daughter.

So I knocked on the bathroom door, and asked my sister the social worker her opinion of my decision. She, at least, would have no ax to grind. To my great dismay, she dismissed my aspirations with an unemotional brevity that had the horrid ring of truth to it. "I think you're nuts!" she said. "Can I borrow your hair dryer?"

But I did have one last ace up my sleeve. There was a kindly psychiatrist in Wilmington for whom I'd been doing some baby-sitting. As he drove me home several nights later, I asked him, cautiously, tentatively, his opinion. By now I had learned to keep my audacious hopes to myself. He was delighted, happy, nonjudgmental, and welcoming. "Of course you'd make a wonderful doctor. Don't be discouraged. Your parents are only concerned that you may get hurt. Study hard, don't give up, keep trying. You have what it takes."

By now I had a perverse need to make sure he understood the reality that all the others had had no trouble grasping. "But I'm not good in science. I have a spider phobia. I don't have enough money. I don't know if I have what it takes to keep going through all those disappointments. If calculators were invented now, I probably wouldn't even know how to use one. I'm Jewish. I'm a girl. I come from a cow college. I like good books, good music, good conversation." I took a deep breath. "I'm a well-rounded human being!"

"Go to it, kid," he said cheerfully. It was all I had to hear. All I needed was one human being to fly with me in the face of all the bitter realities and believe that I could do it. All I needed was one person to help me, and I was ready to take the sour counsel of all the others and turn it to my advantage.

To this day I am convinced that the only reason I got through medical school was to prove to all those people who loved me that they were dead wrong. I became a doctor to spite my parents, my counselors, my teachers, and my friends. I refused to give up because I had to prove that I could do it. I sacrificed many pleasures and satisfactions for the greater happiness of mastering myself, and the lesser happiness of making those near and dear to me eat large portions of uncooked, black-feathered bird. The entire ten-year experience became less the pursuit of medicine than the pursuit of myself. One could say that, in a sense, I did it for the same reason some women abandon long-term marriages —to find myself. The outcome was about what you'd anticipate.

At this point you are expecting me to say that I realize now what a dumb reason I had for going into medicine, that stubborn pride and refusal to quit have nothing to do with being a good doctor. But I am going to surprise you. I think that pride and stubbornness and the refusal to quit are *very good* reasons for pursuing a medical career to the end, certainly as good as the other reasons I've since heard from students. The desire to undertake a killingly difficult regimen, and have something real and concrete to show at the end, is no less valid than the vague and mushy desire "to help people" or "to conquer disease." The savage will to victory is no less important than curiosity to understand pathological processes. It is certainly more honest than entering a profession to "do good" with a naiveté that blinds the student to the realization that much of medicine is a very dirty business, indeed. Furthermore, it is better than undertaking this course of study because one has been *programmed* to do it by ambitious parents who want their kids to have the most prestigious profession our country still has to offer. The concept of conquering medicine because, like the mountain, it is there represents the highest ideal of adolescent striving, and generates precisely the kind of fervor that is *required* by the study of medicine. No one should undertake it who doesn't want it more than anything else in the world.

Let's talk about this some more later on, but for the moment let me just say that I believe that there is an element of "I can't give up, I won't give up" in every person who eventually receives a medical diploma. I may have possessed it to an exaggerated extent, but it is a common denominator, a recurrent theme that runs through everyone who chooses this road and runs it through to the bloody end. If you don't have it, thank your lucky stars and be a credit to some other profession.

I will not feel bad if you walk away from it, nor would old counseling pros like my cousin Milton. He knew that people who cannot fight to exhaustion to overcome the seemingly insurmountable task of getting into medical school will not know how to fight to preserve those patients whose prospects are as bleak, or the integrity of their profession when it is assaulted. People who have achieved easily tend to expect as their due what life often will not or cannot bring them, and they are then ill-equipped to handle the resultant resentment and frustration. "It takes a tough man to make a tender chicken." And, in a sense, it takes a tough training to make a tender doctor.

When I graduated from medical school, the first lap of my training completed, Milton, grinning from ear to ear, came in from Brooklyn with his wife. (Six months later he was dead, another cardiologist whose skill could not save him from his own fatal coronary disease.) My parents also came, my mother dropping her voice back down two octaves to refer to me with well-concealed pride as, "My daughter the doctor."

After the exercises were over, we all went out to lunch at a nearby restaurant. At the next table, through sheer blind luck, sat the guidance counselor who had told me seven years before that I'd never get into medical school and that I'd never make it through if I did. I was too much of a lady to do more than shake my still-warm diploma in the general direction of his *boeuf bourguignon.*

Although this book is not an autobiography, I recognize that some of my experiences can be of use to individuals who are seriously contemplating becoming doctors, and who can learn on an intimate level from examining the lives of those who have preceded them. Therefore, if they are not too personal, I am willing to share them. There was a time when I considered my own story to be so atypical as to be worthless to those seeking guidance. But in 1977 I began to write a monthly column for a medical magazine for young medical students, recent graduates, and the academic faculty who taught them. In this series, I discussed incidentally many of the traumatic remembrances of my medical education, seeking no less to unburden myself than to inspire others to work toward a more humane ideal. To my complete surprise and lurid fascination, I found that my experiences had *not* been all that unusual, nor were they as dated as I would have been the first to suppose. Whenever I did my audience the courtesy of apologizing for referring to some relic of an incident that had happened to me fifteen years before, I received letters from people across the country assuring me that my perceptions were not only contemporary but as common as ever. My column almost became a game of one-upmanship, in which readers invariably wrote to say, "Hey, you think what happened to you is mind-blowing? Let me tell you what happened to me in anatomy class yesterday!" These

letters, some of which I will be sharing with you, convinced me
that medical education, for all its recent upheavals in curriculum,
affirmative action, and philosophy, was still basically a love-hate
affair between raw recruits and their master sergeants.

What also became increasingly clear was that many of my
readers had known very well what it was to be a doctor, but had
not known what is was to *become* one. Most had no realistic
appreciation of what the prolonged medical-educational experience was going to be like until they were knee deep in it, and in
no position to stop the process if they wanted to get off. A number,
like me, had wanted to be doctors so badly they were willing to
undertake it blindly, and then do *anything* without question, until
the ultimate moment of release. Saddest of the letter writers were
those who had matured late in their studies and regretted their
decision to study medicine, but who had so much invested in their
status they literally could not break away without calling down
on their heads an intolerable amount of abuse from family, society,
and conscience.

After forty-eight months of a startingly intimate dialogue with
students and teachers through these columns, I suppose it was
natural that I would want to write a book that would help prospective physicians evaluate realistically the twelve-year odyssey upon
which they wanted to embark. A great deal had been written and
played out in support of the physician mystique; the experience of
medical education, however, was not so highly mythologized. It
seemed to me that the opportunities for creative intervention
would be greatest at the beginning of the adventure.

The big challenge, of course, would be to convey "the thrill of
victory" and "the agony of defeat" equally, in tempered, reasoned
dosages. It requires great skill, I am finding out, to tread the fine
line between preparing people adequately for a tough but exhilarating experience, and scaring the hell out of them. Like Milton,
I feel obligated to be realistic and tell the truth in this volume.
But how can one subjective individual know what the truth really
is? And doesn't every reader make his or her own truth, from the

same set of facts, as I once had with Milton? And is now the right time for you to hear it? I believe so or, like Milton, I'd send you back home on the Pennsylvania Railroad with much of the great unknown still unknown. I, like many doctors, have always hated the unknown and do not see much value in it.

So, since it is impossible for me to be objective, I will do the next best thing. I will try to be fair. I will tell you what I know and what I have seen, and will respect your ability to form your own conclusions. I will try to keep from preaching or offering advice in areas where only you can make a decision. I will try to be helpful, so you can read and gather impressions that will contribute to an informed career decision. I will pray that my material is powerful enough to attract those of you who are undecided and would make the kind of superb physicians our profession needs. I will also hope that it will turn none of this same population away, for I care deeply about the future of medicine, and want only the finest human beings to enter it.

Occasionally I will make reference to a book or article on the subject of choosing medicine as a career, and I will tell you why I think you should read it. There is a growing literature, and most of it is fascinating. None of it can substitute for what your inner spirit tells you, but the more you learn about yourself and others like you, the more use you will eventually be to those you wish to help.

Credibility demands that you know something about me. Perhaps some of you know me from the articles I referred to in *Medical Dimensions* and *The New Physician*; it is possible but not likely. I am a doctor who chose to specialize in social medicine and community health because, as much as I loved taking care of patients, I felt that I could serve them better, and make best use of my talents, working on the community level. I have been a health commissioner, a hospital departmental director, a clinician in a state mental hospital, and a teacher of residents in primary care.

All of medicine involves giving up things that you like to do in order to become more proficient at something else. The thing that I hated to give up the very most was delivering babies. I had about seventy babies before my internship year was over, and every one was such a high, none can be forgotten. It was worth going to medical school just to help a woman push.

As you have already discerned by now, I am a pretty candid person, no longer overly impressed with authority or power. I don't pussyfoot and I don't beat around the bush. (I *do* succumb occasionally to clichés.) I have an irrepressible and ridiculous sense of humor, which I often use to make very serious points. I have a special eye for the idiosyncrasies and foibles of doctors and the community in which they practice; most of my articles have been satire dealing with the social problems of medical practice in the United States today. I also tend to assume that most people mean well until proven otherwise, but I am capable of being utterly wicked to people who deserve it. And I care very much about *you*.

Now let's go on and talk some more about what it means to become a doctor, what the experience is like, what accommodations have to be made, and how the joys and terrors balance out.

2.
A Very
Nosy Question

The first question that the new pre-med will encounter is, simply, "Why do you want to be a doctor?" It is also the most frequent, recurring hundreds of times before the respondent is a free agent and able to tell nosy "buttinskys" to mind their own business. Although the question may seem straightforward enough, it is actually a deeply personal inquiry that often represents an unnecessary intrusion into the victim's private world. That is why people may feel an instinctive reluctance to answer this question and even experience a sense of embarrassment about the whole business. For some, it is like being asked to discuss why they believe in God. In point of fact, few people handle it very well at all. What can one say? Everything sounds so trite and sentimental, so stilted and self-conscious:

> Ever since I was a little tyke I have cut up worms to see what they look like inside.

> I have always wanted to take care of sick people.

> My mother died of cancer, and I vowed that someday I would help people like her.

My guidance counselor told me that I was good in math and science and poor in verbal abilities, so I should become a doctor.

I was sick once as a kid, and when the doctor came, he let me play with his silver watch, and ever since . . .

I must admit, however, that answers are becoming more imaginative and varied nowadays:

My shrink thought it would be a good way for me to get rid of my spider phobias.

After I left my husband and the four kids, I promised myself I would do what I'd always wanted to do through all those twenty long years of marriage to a man who ran around with other women after I gave up my career to put him through school.

My country has sent me to study medicine, as we have only one physician to every 687,923 persons in the mountain regions.

My father said if I didn't do this, I'd have to go into the family business [ladies' dry goods].

My father always wanted me to be a doctor; he's a plumber, and he has money, but he wants a diploma in the family.

My brother got a Ph.D. in English and he's driving a cab, and my sister got a Ph.D. in history and she's taking in washing . . . .

I have been toying with the idea of starting a neo-Marxist economic revolution in this country, and I need an indisputable power base from which to launch it.

I'm Jewish.

I want ultimately to do molecular biochemical engineering research at the postgraduate level, and I've been advised that medicine is the least crowded and least competitive field from which to enter it.

I had a vision in the middle of the night, and my roommate thought I was drunk.

I feel that women (Chinese, minorities, migrants, etc.) should be given the opportunity to consult physicians who are women (Chinese, minorities, migrants, etc.).

I have been programmed since birth by my overly ambitious parents to become a surgeon in a lucra-tive subspecialty, and I am going along with it as they are probably right and I wish to delay my adolescent rebellion for a while longer.

Well, some of the above reasons may be a bit exaggerated. But what can you say to that awful question, "*Why do you want to be a doctor?*"

I am willing to bet that most answers given to this ritualized question constitute social facade, and that not only do most people not know why they want to be doctors, if they did know, they probably wouldn't like it very much. It is important to realize that people who elect to spend their lives dealing with death, torment, human suffering, slimy bodily organs and their even more slippery periodic and aberrant excreta, have agenda that lie too deep for foolish questions and too complex for facile resolu-tion. Most people don't know why they wanted to be doctors until they are old enough to be their own grandparents, and that is probably nature being merciful in the extreme.

Besides, the question is imprecise and serves only to highlight the anxiety of the examiners lest they let the wrong sort into the profession! What people really wish to know is not a person's ultimate *motivation* (*Why* do you want to be a doctor?), but their ultimate *performance* (Are you going to be a *good* doctor?). They would be better off asking a more objective and structured question like, "Why do you think that medicine is the right choice for you?" Although no more enlightening, it is less obnoxious, and would give a more concrete base for the victim to use in fudging answers.

Students being subjected to questions like this should realize, however, that society pours millions of tax dollars into educating each graduate and certainly has the right to know that persons on whom it is extending its largesse will probably complete and make good use of their training. Dropouts cost a fortune. Only in America would students be chosen primarily on how they answered the self-serving question, "What's in it for me in becoming a doctor?" In China, at least until recently, prospective medical students have been chosen by their own comrades on the basis of how well they might serve the people in this particular capacity. It would be nice if we could learn some of this altruism and unemotional functionalism from them, but we probably won't. People who don't know why they wanted to become doctors themselves will persist in torturing the next generation with the same dumb questions. There isn't very much anyone can do about this invasion of privacy but play the game, tell them what they want to hear, and try not to be too sentimental in the response.

Make no mistake. I am not saying that it isn't important to have some real insight into why you want to travel this difficult road. I'm saying only that it is really no one's business but yours, as your motivation, real or perceived, may not be positively correlated with your ultimate performance as a decent, skilled, and compassionate clinician. So, why *do* you want to study medicine? Aside from the fact that, like the mountain, it is there, and there is nothing else in this world that you want to do?

Please think about it, and do it now—this chapter, this page— for once the move is made it is hard to extricate yourself. So much ego becomes invested, so much money, so many familial hopes, so many plans for the future, so many legal and moral commit-ments. I don't know of anyone who has walked out, as a pre-medical student, as a medical student, as an intern or resident, who has not done it after months of moral anguish, paroxysms of guilt, conflicts raging right out there on the surface. Often this is compounded by real feelings of ill-will on the part of people left behind, toward whom reality commitments have been made. It's rough to mend mistakes when you are close to thirty years old.

If at the moment you are unable to articulate a clear reason for your longing, without sounding like a fugitive from the list on the preceding pages, let me "talk around" it a little with you. It may help your thinking.

First, let's dismiss the notion that people study medicine because of a simple complex of talents, attributes, and skills. Take, for example, people who are "good with their hands." When students tell me that they were advised to consider medicine because they were manually dextrous, I wonder why their mentors didn't suggest they turn to the practice of faith healing, which totally substitutes hands for brains. I mean, *really*! More reason-able alternatives for such gifted people include making shell jewelry, doing fine embroidery, the "handyman special" business, dentistry, playing the harp, and executive typing.

People who are good at science, mathematics, engineering, and the like would probably be just as well off going directly into science, mathematics, engineering, or the like. Why medicine?

People who genuinely enjoy caring for others could have excel-lent careers in nursing, social work, the restaurant business, motel management, and psychological counseling.

People who have overwhelming curiosities about nature would no doubt be just as happy in biology, horticulture, dolphin train-ing, or weather divination.

People who wish to be present at critical moments in other people's lives could be just as well satisfied in the ministry, mid-wifery, or grave digging.

People who enjoy grinding out medical and scientific research papers could be copy editors or medical journalists. People who relish medical management could become hospital administrators (or enter an intensive program of psychotherapy!). And people who want to change the health-care status of the country could go to Washington and join the House Ways and Means Committee.

I hope I have made my point, which is that, like a baker's dozen, the sum is more than its component parts. Now that we have ascertained that there is a little of all, or most, of the above in *you*, are you ready to consider an alternative system of motivations that is probably playing a very real part in your decision? As I look at myself, my friends, and my colleagues, a number of these often-hidden motivations seem to become more and more apparent. They may well pertain to you, too. You may not be aware of them, nor will you wish to accept all of them, but I'll roll them out for you anyway.

I suspect that one impelling force in the choice of medicine as a profession is the need to be of service combined with a recognition that the status of this service must not be subservient to others in any way. People who choose medicine like to be masterminds, the overseers, the engineers of service, rather than the humble effectors thereof. They want free, untrammeled rein to do their good, and people to supervise who will help them carry out their therapeutic works. They have a curiosity about the forces of nature and expect a laboratory to help them ferret them out. They have a conviction about how medical care should be disseminated and expect a hospital and/or clinical office to help them deliver it.

Although they would be quick to deny the realization, many are elitists of superior intellectual and social convictions, who find it difficult to talk to others without "talking down." It is for this reason that most physicians, denied the opportunity to study medicine, would not consider nursing or any other "service" profession that could not in some way match the prestige, the glamour, if you will, of medicine. It is for this reason, also, that it is so hard to get physicians to work smoothly in interdisciplinary teams, or even to utilize other health professionals in a properly collegial way.

Although there are definite impediments to having an M.D. after one's name (such as inflated motel bills, unwelcome calls in the middle of the night from strangers passing through, and snide remarks about one's pecuniary status), I know of no physician who has voluntarily renounced his or her two appended initials. Doctors recognize better than anyone else that they occupy a privileged position in society, and most of them feel it's highly deserved. The call to service, but only at the highest administrative level, characterizes most of today's physicians. For better or worse. I say that as much as possible without value judgment. I say that recognizing a lot of it in myself. What kind of a bell does that strike with you? And is it valid?

Another impelling force in the choice of medicine as a profession is the striving toward intellectual acquisition, but only in a field that is essentially unknowable and unconquerable in its totality. Medicine is like a galaxy that can be explored in its sum or in part through light-years, yet always there is something beyond that still cannot be touched. This tantalizing aspect of medical learning is the lure; in its extreme, it is the great Lorelei of researchers. This may seem ironic to those who think that doctors are narrow, boring people who congregate in little in-groups at parties, talking their polysyllabic, neo-Latinate jargon. But knowing more and more about less and less, and tracking it through to its infinite near-end, is part and parcel of the medical experience. Curiosity about the worlds of man and nature is shared by many scientists; only physicians will pursue the course on behalf of man as person and patient. Are you one of them?

The desire for respect and prestige probably plays a greater role in the choice of medicine as a profession than many physicians would wish to acknowledge, particularly those who are unaware of their own feelings of inadequacy and diminished self-esteem. Doctors in this country are still placed upon such a pedestal, probably undeservedly, that it is hard to divorce recognition of this simple fact from one's more altruistic and intellectual strivings. Skeptics will say that doctors are becoming increasingly devalued in this age of malpractice, second opinions, and patient-oriented sunshine laws. That is true. But even as doctors as a group have come under fire, so people tend to cling to their individual physicians, believing that they are the exceptions that prove the rule. The pedestal may be chipped at the base, turning green, and covered with pigeon droppings, but it still stands secure, as does the physician on it. Does that position appeal to you?

Closely allied to the need to be admired, respected, and valued is the need for power. I wonder how many people considering a career of helping people realize that power over the patient's life and death is just a small part of their work? Society has given medical practitioners other far-reaching powers in support of their work. Consider that physicians control who can be employed and who cannot; who can be hired for certain positions and who must be sent away; who can be reimbursed for staggering health-care bills and who may be destroyed financially. They decide who can return to school and who must lie abed. They determine who can live in Boston near the grandchildren, and who must take his sinuses to Arizona. They even decide who is free to travel and who will be grounded.

Consider that a letter to the editor signed with a physician's name carries more weight in the public eye than any other (even when he or she is making some downright opinionated statements that have nothing whatsoever to do with the practice of medicine). Consider the importance of a letter of reference from a physician (particularly to medical school), or the ease with which his or her application for credit is accepted by a tight-fisted, hard-hearted, friendly neighborhood bank. Consider, moreover, that physicians control virtually the entire practice of sick-care management in the country (the money people notwithstanding), setting administrative and professional standards in most health-care institutions.

Any way you look at it, physicians are powerful people, and the way in which they manage this power is a direct function of how much they needed it in the first place. The best physicians are those who have no hang-ups about experiencing or using power, and who accept it as part of the job. If they can't be that grown up, the least we can expect is that they will recognize the need for power in themselves, and do what they can to under-stand it and make it work for them. Where do you stand on that issue?

Identification with revered, older figures who are physicians may be a conscious or unconscious motivating factor in turning toward medicine. It is as good an impetus as any, yet will be only as effective as the student's basic capacity to perform in the chosen field. Many people I know were guided by the image of a real person in their lives and were doubly fortunate to have that person take a real interest in their training and subsequent careers. What do people do, however, who feel the pull toward medicine but have never actually known any doctors who personally inspired them?

There is a great trend now for students to call for "role models" upon whom they can pattern their careers. This call comes most frequently from those who have inadequate sources in real life, figures with whom they can identify. This is especially true of minorities and women. Although superficially it makes perfect sense for a woman, for example, to be able to meet other women physicians and see how they manage their lives and careers, there are nevertheless ominous overtones to the phenomenon. Could it imply in any way that people are afraid to be leaders, and unsure of their own capabilities to make something out of nothing? Does it signify that they have lost the capacity to identify with others who are not of their generation, gender, color, or race? Does it mean that they need to move in a pack in order to accomplish their goals and effect change? As you can see, I am still ambivalent about this developing current. It is too bad that certain individuals always have to be "pioneers," and yet the characteristics necessary to be a pioneer are indispensable for being a good and empathic physician.

Part of me does wish that today's students would just do their own thing, and not have to look to my generation for role models. Perhaps this is because I don't know one woman physician who really feels she is doing a foolproof job of managing her family, her career, and her life. She needs to be setting an example like a moose needs a hat rack. But, of course, she will do it—as well as she does everything!

While we're on the subject of role models, it is obligatory for me to make some comment about the role of the Kildares, Welbys, and other television healers. I won't insult your intelligence by implying that these staged and plastic pushers of "code-blue" carts were your primary role models when you started considering medicine. Still, they exist, and probably are as real and as accurate as highly paid writers can make them.

There is a stereotype in medicine that refers to the "programmed" student. Characteristically, this is the bright, fairly passive young man who has been groomed from infancy for medicine and has been conditioned to this role for so long, he is totally incapable of answering honestly whether or not this is truly what *he* wants. Sometimes the parents are quite right in their judgment that Junior would make a very good doctor, and he never discovers that the idea was not his own. In this case, nothing has been violated but free will and the right of a young person to dawdle, deflect, sniff up the wrong tree, and make some powerful mistakes. In other cases, a poor candidate has obviously slipped through the not-infallible medical admissions net. It is not unheard of for very ambitious parents to facilitate the acceptance of their offspring through very generous donations to the school of their choice. The practice is not common, and meets with great public outrage when exposed, but it has been known to happen. In all these cases, a student may be seen to be functioning as the agent of parents. It seems ridiculous that a motivating factor in the decision to study medicine may be nothing more adult than the desire to please one's parents at any cost. But it happens, and is not so remarkable when we consider what tremendous pressures overly ambitious parents may bring upon their hapless children. If you have reason to suspect that such factors are operating on you, run a mile. Medicine is too costly a prize to bring home to one's parents like a newspaper deposited at their feet by the family dog.

Although few people would admit it, particularly those who are barely aware of it themselves, a well-identified reason for wanting to study medicine is simply the desire for a secure and lucrative income. While few people in our society could be faulted for wanting to invest in a career that will enable them to look forward to an ascendant life-style, there are definite problems in looking to medicine as a source of wealth, not the least of which is that it is a chancy and poor way to find it.

Physicians have a very extended training life, twelve years or longer, during which they are spending money as if it were going out of style and failing to bring much in. They don't begin to recoup the tremendous outlay until they are thirty years of age and deeply in debt (if not financially to banks, then emotionally to parents who have supported them well past the age of childhood). Although once they were free to charge whatever the market would bear with minimal overhead, the steady trend over the past twenty years has been to clip the physician's financial wings. The growth of "third-party payers" who have much invested in keeping prices down; the extraordinary and growing costs of necessary malpractice insurance; the trend toward full-time salaried practice; the growth of peer-influenced groups; and the growing solidification of the national health-insurance movement—all have combined to make the physician think twice before he or she views medicine as the last great frontier of unchecked entrepreneurial activity.

People who want to get rich in today's world probably should do it through promoting rock concerts, bio-medical engineering enterprises, or matrimony to a spouse who is the only child of an aged multimillionaire and on excellent terms with him.

It is my pleasure to report that a growing number of women and minority students are thinking of medicine as a career because they feel that they represent an underserved constituency with whom they closely identify, whose needs they keenly understand, and whose interests they feel impelled to protect. It is wonderful to meet and talk with the most dedicated and impassioned of them, and it is only reluctantly that I would throw out a few words of caution.

First, it is important for such students to want to be doctors first, and to serve their people second. Medicine still must be the first master, and since it is sometimes hard to serve two, people must know very clearly to whom their ultimate allegiance lies. I have seen minority students, for example, torn between their need to retain scientific objectivity and their desire to see their people have all the "advantages" other population groups have. What do they do when their communities clamor for a highly visible and popular "service" that they know in their heart of hearts to be of questionable value? Do they "cop out" or fight the very unpopular battle that may result in their being branded "sell-outs" to the establishment? If people are choosing medicine because it is indeed an excellent power base, let them find another that is even better and leave my profession alone. It has enough problems without alien agents with another agenda.

Such persons must also know that they will be placed under an almost intolerable amount of pressure to make good, not only for themselves, but for those whom they represent. They must be doubly strong, sadly enough, for they will be bearing two burdens. There will often be culture struggles, language problems, educational handicaps to overcome, unpleasant personal encounters, probably money problems. In fact, there will be so many onslaughts, you will be absolutely nuts to undertake it. But if ever we needed potential students not to be dissuaded, now's the time and you are they. You will also be rewarded by being just about the most needed and useful people in the history of this country. If you have only the most tentative interest in medicine, and are browsing in very insecure fashion through this book, please get yourself some good and positive counseling, no matter how improbable this career may feel to you now. If there's any chance you can make it, try to find out *stat*. (*Stat* is Latin medical talk, and it means immediately, right now, get your you-know-what into gear.) *See Chapter Ten.*

When all is said and done, the unconscious reasons for wanting medicine are the most potent of all. We all share an intricate network of reasons for entering this field, based upon our primitive feelings about death, separation, transfiguration through suffering, and the ultimate power of healing and regeneration. I'm not a psychiatrist, and dread getting in over my head talking about sublimation, counter-phobias, and flights into activity. I know only instinctively that entering medicine *is* a way of working out puzzlements and conflicts in these areas, and coming to terms with paradoxes in ways that are given to few laypeople. I suppose this may be the most cogent reason of all for seeing the mountain that to other people simply does not exist. All physicians, in a sense, seek to heal themselves, and in doing so, often heal others as well. And sometimes they don't.

I would like to call to your attention an excellent discussion of the realistic and psychological reasons why some people tend to choose medicine as their career. It sums up much of the research that has been done, and presents it in a very readable and thought-provoking way. The book is entitled *Medical Student: Doctor in the Making.* The chapter to which I am referring is called "The Decision to Become a Doctor." Don't miss it! It can help you tap into some of the unconscious reasons that are motivating you at this point in your life. While they are not presented as reasons *not* to go into medicine, they are meant as food for thought.

Now that we have run through some of the very common reasons for studying medicine. I'd like to come back to something that has been on my mind since the start of this chapter. I'd like to say a word to people who are not still in high school or early college, but are coming to this career decision later in life. A number of you have tried other careers and felt dissatisfied; some of you have postponed medicine, which was the only thing you ever wanted, for other temporary life goals. Some of you only now have the financial and temporal reserves that you need to get started. (One of the women in my class in medical school worked nine years as a teacher simply to save up enough money to go to medical school.)

It is accepted belief that older students are more sober, more serious, more goal-oriented, more knowledgeable of themselves and their motivations, more serious about their studies. I'm sure it is true. Nevertheless, I have seen people coming around the second time who were, if it's possible, even more confused than they were the first time. It was all the more awful because there was so much invested in denying it. It is possible, and even probable, that a person can make the same mistake twice, or, to be more exact, make a second mistake as bad as the first.

I knew a woman in the third year of her residency who, at the age of thirty-seven, was going through a real life-goal crisis. She had been a teacher, had lived in Europe, had dissolved a marriage, spoke three languages, thought that medicine would bring all her many talents together at last and give her a unified life work. It just didn't work. She will probably go on practicing medicine because she has to earn a living, and it is a highly lucrative one. But happy she isn't.

I know another woman who was a film editor for years and decided, after working around, through, and under other doctors for a long period, to become a doctor. She figured she was as smart as they were and her brain was underutilized. She was right. But envy and one-upmanship, and the need to prove one's self at a late date, are really poor grounds for studying medicine. This woman is entitled to her free choice of career, but I am not sure that I would want to be her patient. Ultimately, that's how I judge every physician—would I want to be his or her patient?

Coming back to medicine is a tricky business, particularly as the training period is so long and demanding. However, it definitely can be done. My lab partner in anatomy class was a thirty-five-year-old woman with a Ph.D. in psychology, who wanted to climb higher. She did it, and is a marvelously trained and productive individual. I have known and worked with many like her. As long as there's hope and will, there's a chance. Just be careful. Be very, very careful.

3.
Hustling and Other Grubby Practices

As you already know, not having had the benefit of reading the preceding chapter, I could not have made a very informed decision to study medicine. On the contrary, I succumbed to a sudden vision. I have since learned that this is not uncommon. Many people are suddenly triggered by an unremembered (but emotionally significant) episode that occurred in their lives shortly before their sudden decision. Therefore, I was relatively unprepared for the new world into which I was suddenly plunged. Have a look at it, for it is not very different from what you too can expect!

First, I had to field my share of the why-do-you-want-to-be-a-doctor? questions discussed in the preceding chapter. Some of these came from my former English advisers, who wanted to make sure that I didn't get hurt. Others came from my new pre-med advisers, who wanted to make equally sure that this female aspirant with no credentials would not mess up their university's favorable application/acceptance ratio at medical schools. (Cow colleges being low in the pecking order, they could ill afford to encourage too many the likes of me.)

Next, my familiar geographic base shifted from Hullihen Hall, an ivied neoclassical structure that housed the liberal arts, to its architectural counterpart immediately across the commons, Brown Laboratory, whose ivy quivered under a daily barrage of hydrogen sulfide. It was a very symbolic move.

The population base shifted, too. No longer were there fifteen women to every man in my classes; I became one of three women in lecture halls seating seventy. In both respects, it was as if I'd left college completely to enter the real world. Life became work, grimly pursued, and secondary to no other campus activity. Gone were the marching band, the college newspaper, and leisurely coffees with other slovenly intellectuals in the campus food joint, The Scrounge. Yes, college became a business, not pleasure, and suddenly reality was all that mattered.

It is customary to tell students who show signs of healthy high spirits that they are only able to get away with this kind of behavior because they are still in a protected environment. "You'll see how it is when you get out in the real world," people tell them menacingly, implying that the undergraduate university is one large tree trunk to house a thousand small Peter Pans. Incredibly, this fallacy is perpetuated even among pre-medical and medical students, who are somehow made to feel that they should not complain because their life is unreal and transient. They are given the impression that their training is nothing more than a way station to later functioning in a more authentic situation. This is nonsense. Personally, I never felt the pressure of reality *more* than when I was cramming for an exam whose outcome seemed able to make or break me for all eternity.

A lot of the dreaminess got knocked out of me during the first few months. But I was high with a sense of purpose, so perhaps one dream was able to sustain me during the loss of the other. With or without dreams, people have to function, accomplish, and manipulate their environment to suit their own purposes. In developing my strategies of management, it was important to recognize and understand the new phenomena with which I would have to deal. Everyone else was going through the same bewildering process, even the boys in my class who had known from babyhood that someday they were going to be neuro-surgeons.

As I look back on that experience, I find myself able to isolate and describe a number of attributes of medical education with which you should become familiar. They are:

HUSTLING

THE BLOOD LUST OF COMPETITION

THE ACQUISITION OF LONELINESS

TENACIOUSNESS

SURVIVOR GUILT

THE POSTPONEMENT OF IMMEDIATE GRATIFICATION

OVERCOMING HORROR

THE CONSOLIDATION OF CREDIBILITY

THE TESTING OF ETHICAL VALUES

HIPPOCRATIC BONDING

THE DEVELOPMENT OF ADMINISTRATIVE SKILLS

THE DISPENSATION WITH RELEVANCE

THE NARROWING OF CULTURAL HORIZONS

SENSORY DEPRIVATION AND TEMPORARY REALITY LOSS

THE TRANSIENCE OF EXULTATION

THE ROLLER-COASTER EGO

INTEGRATING YOURSELF

I'll discuss each of these in turn. If, while reading, you feel as if you're drowning, keep your sense of humor and irony and hang in. It all gets better. I promise.

HUSTLING

To survive, first and foremost, pre-medical students must be hustlers. Having been the kind of person who took protective coloring in the crowd for much of my life, one of the hardest things for me to learn was how to hustle. Hustling meant doing

whatever was necessary to become "the firstest with the mostest."
Hustling meant having eyes in the back of your head, ears in the
soles of your feet, and six fingers on each hand. It required a
heightened sensitivity to academic rumors that was akin to clair-
voyance. It meant anticipating every unforeseen occurrence; stalk-
ing prey like a tribal huntsman; psyching out every teacher and
lab assistant; mathematically plotting what would be on every
test, based on past tests, teacher mood, the prevailing winds. It
meant being first at the bookstores, lest supplies be limited. It
meant circling calendars four months in advance of minor holidays.

Hustling meant cultivating classmates, the better to barter
objects, favors, services, information. It meant being prepared, as
no Boy Scout would ever have to be, yet knowing simultaneously
how to bail out when caught *un*prepared. It meant being in three
places at once, and having a book on a chair to reserve your place
in the fourth. It meant planning ahead, while mopping up from
behind. It meant ingratiating yourself with those whom you might
or might not have formerly favored, then feeling sleazy about the
polluted relationship (as well you should). Hustling meant reading
lab experiments in *advance*, so that four-hour filtrations could be
set up the night before. It meant napping on the run and sleeping
sitting up. It meant searching faces and hiding things.

Hustling became for me a way of life that has lasted the better
part of twenty-five years. Sometimes I think only a very severe
and exotic form of transcendental medication could ever break the
back of this phenomenon. It's like being a farm kid who still wakes
up at 4:30 A.M., even though there are no cows in the big city. In
part, the hustling mentality is responsible for the productivity,
goal-orientedness, and multiple accomplishments of physicians. In
part, it is also responsible for their drive, their restless pushing on,
and the way they sometimes make their patients hustle, too.

As I try to understand this characteristic of pre-medical
programs, I wonder if we aren't dealing with a chicken-egg
phenomenon. Do student doctors hustle because they are ambi-

tious, compulsive, driven to excellence, and determined to get ahead? In other words, do they do it because it is in their nature to do it? Or do they do it because they see everyone *else* doing it, and they don't dare get left behind? Sometimes I think our profession should arrange for a nice, bald-pated monk in a saffron robe to sit cross-legged on the demonstration tables of each pre-med lab in the United States, to remind us that there is another world to which hustling will not gain us entrance. The danger with being unable to slow down is that someday we may not be able to forgive patients who don't move as fast as we'd like. And why *should* the patient hustle to fulfill our treatment requirements? He's no fool. Besides, he doesn't have to get into medical school!

THE BLOOD LUST OF COMPETITION

A good healthy competitiveness is part and parcel of the medical persona, mine being manifest at the age of five when I could jump rope better than any girl on the block, and pretty proud of it I was, too. But winning at cards or Indian-wrestling is a transient thing, an occasional moment when the blood and spirits shoot up, and reality as well as state of consciousness are briefly altered. The blood lust of medical competition, on the other hand, is an ongoing state of existence. If innocent competition occasionally causes the blood pressure to rise, we may say that a medical student by comparison suffers from "chronic competitive hypertension." When the chronic competitive blood lust reigns, the so-called "normal" or bell curve on which students are marked can do more to ruin the sleep of pre-medical students than all the late-night studying in the world.

Perhaps you have heard that infamous story of the good old days when medical students, enrolled for their first lecture, are informed by the professor, "Gentlemen! Look to the right of you, and look to the left of you. One of you won't be here next term!"

Although medical schools actually have a tremendous financial investment in not flunking out any of the candidates they have selected, students can never bring themselves to believe this. The fear of failure and the rabid desire to do anything in the world to prevent it are two motives that make the pre-medical student one of the most competitive animals in captivity. When one of those mythical three bites that dust, it sure isn't going to be *numero uno*.

I personally did not feel this particular scourge until I arrived at medical school itself, more naive than I had any right to be. The men with whom I worked as an undergraduate actually took pity on me, and made me their mascot. They would keep me up all night, plying me with caffeine and forcing me to spit back all the organic chemistry formulas I thought I would never get through my thick skull. Perhaps they thought it cute that a girl was studying medicine, or perhaps they just liked me. I certainly liked them, and hope they all made it into medical school in the end. They proved that there were isolated pockets of human kindness in the rat race, and that people under stress can retain their humanity.

THE ACQUISITION OF LONELINESS

There is a unique loneliness in being a medical student, and it is a vital forerunner of the aloneness that follows into later years. It is not all that unpleasant, merely a sense that there is a world into which you are being drawn, and to which you cannot bring even your nearest and dearest. It is a fundamental separation, in which books, facts, learning processes, and experiences become close companions, and the friends of before recede somewhat.

I'm not sure why I refer to this loneliness as acquired. I guess on some level I do see it as a robe that must be picked up, put around one's shoulders, and made one's own by a very active process. Loneliness doesn't just *happen* to you by a passive osmosis. It is something you work at in some crazy way. It is also manifest in sudden, veiled ways.

You are aware of it the first time you see or do something that upsets you, and you feel instinctively that this is something you must deal with without sharing it. Perhaps you sense that the subject is taboo in ordinary conversation, or it is something that others will just not want to hear. Perhaps you are wrong, but something says, "Spare your friend. Don't tell her. She wouldn't understand, nor is it necessary for her to understand. First try to understand it yourself." As I said, perhaps you were wrong. Your friend may be sensitive to your distress and want very much to discuss it with you. But your judgment is not what concerns us here, only the voice that tells you to maintain your silence. It is very real.

There is a clear distinction between this acquired loneliness and the real loss of friends and sweethearts who cannot withstand the competitive assault of your studies. Some will leave you cold, in which case you have not lost much of value. Others remain your friends, but the bonds are inevitably strained, as you find yourself unable to be available as a true friend should be. You may think that you are sacrificing only yourself and for yourself when you begin your studies, but you are also punishing those who have come to need you, use you, share with you, and look to you for the rights and "perks" of friendship. Of course, you are developing new relationships among all those who are in this with you (including those who inspire your blood-lust competitiveness), but they are a highly specific group. What of the others?

"Finking" on friends is an awful feeling, and was one of the things I had the most trouble with when I took my big plunge. I was such a typically unyielding, obsessive-compulsive student, I would have watched my own house burn down if calling the fire department would have interrupted my studies. I remember when one of my closest friends called to tell me that she was eloping to Elkton (the local quick-marriage town) and that, if I hurried, I could be her companion at the biggest moment of her life. I knew how much it meant to her, for she had met her guy in my living room. But she got married without me. Of course it scarred the friendship; it *had* to. And this was not an isolated instance.

Still, what do you do when something important happens, and you have an exam the next day?

TENACIOUSNESS

Remember that old joke about the guy with the violin who grabs an old man on the subway and asks him, "How do you get to Carnegie Hall?" and the old man says sagely, "Practice, my son, practice!" If you asked the same instructions to medical school, the old man would probably say, "Hang in, my son, hang in!"

For every genius who intimidates all the other members of the class, there are a hundred students who gain admission to medical school by simply refusing to go away. The truth is that the ability to plod like a blinded ox pulling a millstone is probably the single most valuable attribute a student can develop. The ability to pick oneself up after a mortal blow like a failing grade on a quiz is as necessary as breathing. Since faculty and administration will be ever present to remind the student of his or her lowliness, there is no point in joining the chorus. Although anyone can keep going when things are moving right, it takes a very special masochistic skill to continue to offer cheek after cheek when things are going wrong. A real pre-med simply can't run out of cheeks. Nor can he or she run out of two legs to stand on, or a well-cushioned butt to sit on for more study.

Getting an important point across can mean repetition (as you will learn when you instruct patients in how to prepare for a barium emema), so let me say it again. *It is impossible to give up!* Most people who don't make it to medical school are people who've given up, in person, fact, or spirit. Another image comes to my mind, which is in itself a sad commentary on what the regimen requires. I see a punch-drunk fighter in a ring, bloody and battered, hearing bells and coming back for more. I hate myself for that graphic image, but it's there and I won't censor it. Besides, *Rocky* had a happy ending, didn't it?

Sir William Osler, who wrote a number of classical pieces for medical students, including *Aequanimitas and Other Essays*, suggested that they live life in day-tight compartments, the way ships functioned with watertight compartments. *"What each day needs, that shalt though ask, each day will set its proper task. . . ."*

There are definite advantages to living one day at a time, hard as this may be for the Type A personality to believe. It is easier to hang in if one has only to get through one day at a time. This reduces *anticipatory dread*, the great plague of students under pressure, and helps to limit trauma to the amount a student can handle at any one given point. "He who fights and runs away, lives to fight another day." Osler probably didn't say that, but he should have. There are days when you just can't hack certain chores, and there's no point in forcing what may come naturally at another, more opportune time.

Living a day at a time, apportioning your battles, and helping yourself as much as possible greatly facilitate the attainment of a long-range goal. So, if you want to be a doctor, hang in. It may not get you to Carnegie Hall. But it will certainly help you to get to the bedside.

SURVIVOR GUILT

Survivor guilt refers to the pain that sensitive people feel when they alone achieve a goal once shared by close associates now lost. Most people associate this phenomenon with the nightmares of those who have crept out of death camps, burning tenements, and lifeboats from ships lost at sea. My first experience with this was with a woman classmate named Anna. She was a dark-haired, pretty girl with a foreign accent, who loved parties and clothes, and floated along like a waterlily on a large pond of male chemistry majors. I was delighted to have her around, in part because she validated my desire, as a woman, to become a physician. I loved her breezy ideas, born of a sympathetic European attitude toward women in medicine, regarding the compatibility of minimal study with the achievement of goals. Unfortunately, she flunked out.

On some level I must have known that she wasn't studying enough and was having too much fun to be a successful pre-medical student, but the shock and horror of losing her made me feel unworthy, marked, and more vulnerable than ever. I reacted as John Wayne would have done. It was like watching a comrade fall in the desert, then stripping her boots and her canteen and walking out toward the horizon. My stoicism tells me that I must have been denying the threat to myself. After all, she was a woman who had unsuccessfully tried to prove that you could be a woman *and* a doctor, too. All I know is that the following semester there were only two women left. One of the three had fallen.

Although I didn't know what the term "survival guilt" meant until six years later, it was not the first time I was to experience it. My freshman chemistry partner in medical school also bit the dust and went home to Kentucky. Another classmate committed suicide shortly after graduation. And think how many women graduates fell simply because they wanted to raise their kids the traditional way—with a mommy at home while they were young!

THE POSTPONEMENT OF IMMEDIATE GRATIFICATION

Serious students have to be able to postpone their needs for immediate gratification if they are to succeed. Of course, if they're not *getting* any immediate gratification, not much has been lost. Very often when people are in a position to expect having to give things up, they tend to idealize and exaggerate the loss. It's really a form of self-flattery.

At times like this, students are prey to the belief that while they are locked in doing their drone number, the rest of the world is out there getting theirs. It's hard to be locked up on a gorgeous October day with forty-seven pounds of textbooks, while everyone else is raking piles of leaves or carrying blankets down to the bleachers for a home game. Most of this ideation is masochistic self-torture and doesn't last long, fortunately.

The truth of the matter is that pre-medical students soon become masters at the art of condensing work to fit the time allotted, and budgeting their stolen fun in a way that makes it twice as enjoyable. They learn how to sample pleasures, how to provide substitutes for them, or, when all else fails, how to go on the binge to end all binges that lasts them through another month of grind.

The ideal of the bookworm is no longer valued in the eighties, and no points are racked up by professional slaves. If anything, students are encouraged to live as normal a life as possible. Unfortunately, no one has lowered either the work loads or the demands for excellence of performance, and in the words of the old song, "Something's gotta give . . ." If you follow the iron-clad rules of hustling, it will probably be whatever is least beneficial to you in the long run—like food, rest, and periodic trips to the bathroom!

Since, as has been observed, pre-meds tend to be compulsive types, who worry things to death and gnaw on facts like rats eat hard cheese, it actually takes tremendous self-discipline to make sure that the books are set aside long enough to really unwind. Medical school deans will tell you that their greatest problems with over-zealous medical students involve getting them to loosen up and recognize that they can't possibly learn *everything*. Sooner or later they have to have the capacity to say, "Enough is enough." I suppose one of a student's major challenges is to be able to walk away from a half-finished task and still have a good time, free of guilt, free of the nagging doubt that he or she should be somewhere else, free of the torment that maybe this time the exam will be devoted exclusively to what was skipped because of the spur-of-the-moment beer at the local joint. It's all part of the "psyche 'em out" game, and anyone who can hustle and manage the blood-lust competition can certainly handle the "immediate gratification" challenge.

What people don't know is that there are tremendous rewards as the fruits of postponement start to come in. These take the form of pleasing grades; feelings of mastery over very difficult material; the knowledge that requirements are fulfilled, carrying one closer to the ultimate goal; and the revelation that one has really been the master of one's own destiny. Much of my work as an English major was fluff and cotton candy. But there's nothing like a good hard piece of cheese!

OVERCOMING HORROR

For the medical student, the paradigm of the horror experience is the dissection of the cadaver, and we will have more to say about that later. My own nemesis proved to be the humble frog, whose brain I was required to pierce with a needle one day in biology class. To put it mildly, I thought I would die. It was such a seriously traumatic event for me, I really came close to giving up. Not only was it hard for me to believe that someone actually expected me to decerebrate one of God's living creatures, who had done me no harm, but that I was actually expected to *handle* that loathsome, slippery creature as well. I cringed as it leaped around on its cardboard platter.

I will never know why people say they "get sick at the sight of blood" and then think nothing of going out and pithing a frog. I raced to the phone booth and called the psychiatrist in Wilmington. I guess on some level I recognized that psychiatrists knew something about the management of the feelings aroused by frog-pithing. My heart pounded as I wailed into the phone, "I can't, I just can't, no way, I'll die first." "What's the matter?" he asked. "Are you afraid of getting aggressive to a frog?" I hung up and listened to the nickel clunk into the bottom of the box. I had no choice. I went back to the lab, my neck twitching. If I did it, I have no remembrance. But somehow I got through the session. I celebrated it in my sonnet class the next week. I'm sure the shrinks have a good word for the process that enabled me to turn a nightmare into a joke. Here it is. Note the rhyme scheme: *abab, cdcd, efef, gg*. It is a traditional Elizabethan sonnet, in iambic pentameter, entitled "Pippa (Raniens) Passes":

> Last week in lab we butchered up a frog
> In pieces fine as for a dainty stew
> (Experimental creatures like the dog
> For amateurish slicing are too few).
> Before us on a pin-pricked cardboard platter
> Lay a female, belly stuffed wide
> With eggs and things pertaining to that matter
> Which delicacy bids me not confide.
> With forceps fine and scissor snips galore
> Removed were the messy frog entrails
> Whilst formalin and rivulets of gore
> Did not us spare the nauseous details.
> Oh, wretched toad, I thought, with boundless wit
> A sonnet to your graces should be writ!

Experimentation on animals is a necessary part of the learning experience, and those who do not recoil when handling white rats are devoutly to be envied. I don't know what the answer is, or what the best "toughening" process should be. Medicine requires sensitive people who wish to spare patients pain and suffering, and then it forces them to go out and do things that are antithetical to everything they stand for, in the name of science and the scientific method. It is too bad that so often people are left to work out their horror in whatever way they can. Personal resources are often inadequate to the task, and surprisingly in people who would make good doctors. Over and over again, student practitioners are called upon to harness, tame, and stomp on their natural impulses, and if the job is done too severely, there may be unpleasant aftereffects as people become hardened and calloused.

Students should really be encouraged to form support groups on the undergraduate level, to explore honestly what they are going through, and to share the pain with others. Those who have less trouble dealing with these things might be able to serve as a source of strength and consolation to others for whom these violent acts are heavily symbolic and inclined to be traumatic.

It is not always easy to predict when, or how often, the phantom of horror will strike. I was certain that I would have troubles in comparative anatomy, for I love cats and don't like to see them stiff and dead, with great wads of padding forcing their jaws permanently open. But instead I was suffused with the gallows humor so common to students of death, and ended up carrying my kitty home in a great plastic shopping bag to dissect in the basement. My mama, whose feelings about cats were about on par with her feelings about my career choice, couldn't do wash for a week.

It must also be pointed out, to cheer up those who anticipate they might have troubles in this area, that familiarity breeds contempt. The first experiences are the hardest. By the time I was ready to approach my cadaver, it was with a calm heart and a calculating eye. I really did not suffer at all.

We'll have other opportunities to consider this subject.

THE CONSOLIDATION OF CREDIBILITY

One would think that anyone bright enough to maintain a 3.5 index or better, while still making obeisance to the laws of bloodlust competition and hustling, would have no further need to prove fitness for medicine. But no such luck. One of the grubbiest, downright tackiest maneuvers that pre-medical students have been forced to indulge in is the *consolidation of credibility*. Here's why.

Somewhere back in the Middle Ages of medical school entrance procedures, only science students obtained easy acceptance. Then word got out that the power structure wanted "well-rounded individuals," and a few of the unwary raced over to the liberal arts. It soon became apparent, however, that medical schools *lied* when they said that they wanted people who valued the acquisition of foreign languages, courses in belles lettres, and Asian history. While giving lip service to the desirability of the well-rounded person, they went right ahead giving preference to the bio and zoo majors. Those who had fallen into the bear trap of believing the medical schools found themselves stuck up a very tall tree.

When the new word came down that medical school admissions committees were not to be trusted, it became apparent that extracurricular activity to supplement the science major was the only way to go. People had to "consolidate their credibility" by developing all aspects of their personality. When I read the résumés of aggressive people applying to medical school, I can't believe the extent of the extracurricular projects they claim to have experienced. It isn't enough just to be a good student anymore. Nowadays, you must also spend your summers, weekends, evenings, holidays, and several full nights a week consolidating your credibility with such items as:

> Working as an orderly in a hospital or working as a lab technician in a lab

> Working as a candy striper (or gray lady or black belt) in a health center

> Flying back and forth to deepest, darkest Africa as a part-time Peace Corps volunteer

> Building your own home chemistry laboratory and discovering a new enzyme

> Helping a distinguished scientist make a discovery that he can publish before someone else does

Spending the summer as a counselor in a camp for children who are as disturbed as you are

Going to Outward Bound off the coast of Mexico, where you are required to survive for two weeks with nothing but a can of sardines and two bent forks

Doing a survey of the nation's attitudes toward the mental anguish of pre-medical students

Working for the election campaign of a candidate who stands firmly behind increased federal aid for medical education and research

Being a tutor for brain-damaged kids who cannot read but have an uncanny ability to know what day of the week November 13, 2416, will fall on

Building an addition to your parents' home with your bare hands, including plumbing, wiring, carpentry, and interior design.

One would suspect from reading these frantic efforts to impress committees with well-roundedness that not one student in a million knew what it was to lie on his or her back all day and count cumulonimbus clouds crossing the sun. Too bad! What have we done, as a profession, to be so inundated with these damned overachievers?

THE TESTING OF ETHICAL VALUES

We should now discuss a subject for which I do not see any answers at the moment. I am referring to the tremendous ethical dilemmas facing today's pre-medical student, primarily in response to the pressures involved in securing that all-important acceptance to medical school. It has *always* been tough to get in, and if you are a woman or Oriental or black, in many schools your chances now are better than they ever were before. Nevertheless, there are still five or ten applicants for each position and no one knows better than you how unworthy you are to be the one chosen. How far *would* you go to get into medical school?

In order to get in, you have to work hard, get good grades, consolidate your credibility, perfect your hustling methodology, overcome your horror and survivor guilt, deal with the blood lust of competition, maintain your sanity in the face of uncertainty, acquire a little productive loneliness, and . . . be prepared to do a little radical and reconstructive surgery on your ethical values? You heard me. You have to be prepared to make some hard decisions.

I'm not talking about cheating on tests, or fudging lab notes. That's too easy. I'm talking about less obvious decisions, where you are gradually co-opted rather than overtly seduced, where no one knows or cares what you are doing but you yourself. I'm talking about situations where the questionable activity has become so much the norm, so routinized, that one is hard-pressed even to recall why it was once considered unworthy. The "slippery slope" of the pre-med life can produce a thoroughly sophisticated, incredibly cynical, vigorously well-defended, sincerely unethical person in no time flat. *I would even go so far as to say that it is impossible to be a graduate of an American medical school and still be a completely moral person.*

I'll give a few examples. Let's say that you are tempted by a course entitled "Russian History from Peter the Great to Catherine the Great: A Cultural, Intellectual, and Economic Study." (That's actually a bad example, since it happened to be a dull time in Russian history, but never mind.) Your grandfather was Russian, and you have always been fascinated by the subject. A little inquiry reveals that the teacher is one of those marvelous old martinets whose students adore him even as he works them into the ground. Moreover, he still thinks an A in a course should be a reflection of A work. If you take the course, you risk serious damage to your overall grade index.

On the other hand, the same time slot offers "Principles of Phonetic Speech." It includes a history of the life of George Bernard Shaw, the reading of a translation of *Major Barbara* into phonetic alphabet, and a six-week workshop on voice projection and the art of mellifluous speech. (Don't laugh, please, I once took this course.) You are guaranteed an A because the instructor is so hard up for candidates you can literally make your own deal with him in advance, including a schedule of acceptable no-shows. You will have done your index an immeasurable good turn—sort of like a tetanus booster after you've stepped on a rusty nail.

Which do you pick? Why? Can you see a moral dilemma in this situation? How many of you would pick the latter, promising yourselves that someday you will get a good book on Russian history and educate yourselves, without "wasting time" going to formal classes? Yes, precisely. Just as we would have expected. Well, don't blame yourselves too much. All's fair in love and war. I might have done the same thing myself.

Here's another situation. All of you have been haunting the old fraternity files for copies of the histology exam for the past ten years. The guy who runs the course usually asks the same kinds of questions and the test is always lengthy and detailed. When you arrive for the exam, you discover, to your horror, that this time the dumb bunny hasn't even changed it at all! He's lazier than you are, and has slipped you last year's word-for-word quiz! Do you say, "Hey, buddy, this is an insult and you have been disrespectful of your students"? Or do you shut your mouth and answer the questions by rote, sitting there the full hour so that he doesn't suspect the source of your confusion? Do you tell yourself that if you say anything, you'll get everyone *else* in trouble? Do you tell yourself that it is just a dumb histology exam and you knew it all, anyway, and besides, since when do exams ever test how much a person knows about a subject? Do you remind yourself that this is all *his* fault? Congratulations! You have reacted in fairly standard fashion to the idiocy of the system.

Let's say one of your required readings is an article in *The New England Journal of Medicine*. The library has a reference copy that is "on hold" for all ten members of your section. As a hustler, you are the first there. It is a wonderful article. When you are done, do you quietly, and without leaving a trace, remove the article from its page with a pocket razor, so that no one else will be able to have access to it before the exam? What? You wouldn't do such a thing? Your buddies would. Ask any medical librarian what major journals end up looking like before a big exam.

Still another area of ethical testing is starting to emerge in the repayment of educational loans contracted by students during their long tenure in school. The average indebted pre-med piles up many thousands of dollars in loans by the time the training period is over and immediate repayment begins. Although repayment seems far away to the college freshman, the day of reckoning eventually arrives and, according to the federal government, doctors (and lawyers, too) are among their biggest deadbeats. As hard as it is to believe, a number of "head-hunting" agencies have been established across the United States to try to track down those who have walked out on their obligations, despite their entrance into a lucrative profession.

I cannot share the reasons for these defaults with you, because I just don't understand them myself. Reason tells me that there must be a plausible excuse, probably related to the sheer immensity of the debt, and the need to have some release of obligation after so many years of another kind of servitude. But it still doesn't add up very well. You might want to consider these temptations as real ones that you may someday face, even as you take the first financing steps as an undergraduate.

The entire emerging world of bio-medical ethics, which in the past concerned only those engaged in certain forms of human experimentation and extreme therapies, now covers much of the medical world and the pre-medical world as well. Before we can have "medical ethics," we have to have a high level of "personal morality." How's yours?

HIPPOCRATIC BONDING

A rather curious relationship tends to develop between premedical students. In many ways it resembles the mutual clinging and interdependence of two soldiers on their own in a foxhole under enemy fire. They rely upon each other for security and solidarity in the fight, and they mooch each other's cigarettes and cookies from home. Yet, remember, we have talked about the blood-lust competition of medical students. Who else are they beating out for the valued place in the incoming freshman class but these very same buddies of the trenches? Students lead a very schizophrenic existence. They are forced to provide aid and sustenance to their competitor in order to retain their own stability and humanity, and then they must suffer when that same person turns up with a higher grade on an exam. The scenes when grades and end-term reports are in remind me of what takes place when a young woman must congratulate her best friend on being asked to the prom by the local football hero, while she still waits for the phone call that may not come. True compassion does spring through, however, and then genuine joy that another has succeeded. Medical students know how to identify with each other, and they recognize that they are all very much in it together.

These feelings are solidified and strengthened during the coming years in medical school and the many years of practice that follow. The close-knit bonding of physicians is legendary in our society. Just ask a few plaintiffs in malpractice suits, who claim that they can never get a doctor to testify against another doctor.

Many doctors feel unable to explain to the outside world the strength of the bond that ties them, no matter what their personal opinions might be about the way cases are being managed. They belong to a great fraternity that has gone through traumatic long wars together, and they believe that no one else could possibly appreciate what it was they endured.

I know that for many years I felt that way myself. Perhaps the feeling sprang from the loneliness I spoke of earlier, when I first realized that there were things that "were not to be spoken of abroad," as the Hippocratic oath quaintly puts it. It seemed that nothing could match the uniqueness of our educational experiences. But some of that feeling has since diminished. Recognition has come that there are people in other professions who have felt that overwhelming sense of responsibility for human life, people like airplane pilots, nuclear physicists, even air traffic controllers and firemen. Ours is not the only bonding, and in fact it may be a rather chauvinistic and "counterproductive" one at that. People who feel that only a select in-group can appreciate the feelings they keep locked up are not really free to develop close relationships with others, not even those in the best position to empathize—like spouses, nurses, and *patients themselves!*

I once wrote an article comparing doctors and the firemen for whom I once worked in Los Angeles. I tried to examine how these two groups of death-facing, closely knit workers handled their love relationships with each other. I called it "Fire and Ice." You'd be surprised what differences there are in the ways people under tension care for one another.

4.
The Chapter
I Didn't Mean
to Write

Center Barnstead, New Hampshire

August 22, 4:45 A.M.

I did not intend to write this chapter, but it occurs to me that the experience that prompted it might be of use to you. But first, let me set a scene for you.

I am typing this at a very rickety small table purchased at auction several days ago, in the country kitchen of my old farmhouse in New England. I came up here to my hideaway to try to get this book started during a few precious, uninterrupted vacation days. My husband is at home with the cats, and the neighbors have been warned to leave me be. Obligingly, the weather has cooperated by pouring down rain and fog for three days running.

It has been wonderful to be able to do something, for once in my life, without having to do a million other things at the same time. When I went to bed last night, I noted with the satisfaction of an experienced hustler that I had accomplished fifty type-written pages in three days, and for the first time permitted myself to wonder if what I had written was good enough. For many physicians, *nothing* is ever good enough, and I did not spare myself some agony about the probable uselessness of my growing book. In particular, I wondered if I'd been too hard on you, if I'd been too negative in my approach and not emphasized enough of the "positives" along with the problems. I resolved to make sure that before this book was done there would be no doubt in anyone's mind that I thought that medicine could be unparalleled fun and the chance of a lifetime for people who wanted to have a positive influence in this world.

It also seemed to me that I had not handled sufficiently well the short section dealing with the unconscious motives people had for choosing medicine. Milton had been easy on me. So why wasn't I being easy on you? In the name of honesty, was I ramming some painful information down your throats for sadistic reasons of my own? Was there a part of me that may have actually *enjoyed* notifying young people of the rough years ahead? After all, older doctors are notorious for wanting young interns and residents to suffer as they did, not sleeping enough, not being paid enough, doing a lot of "scutwork." I had never counted myself among them, but we all do have an unconscious mind that can play tricks on us if we are not careful. I went to sleep thinking these thoughts and listening to the rain.

Unexpectedly, I had a frightening nightmare just a few moments ago. I have not had such a bad dream in a number of years. As I awoke, it seemed to me that I was quite hot, and as I groped to turn on the light, I recognized that the electric blanket, set to an all-time high of ten, coupled with the heavy quilt I'd thrown over my frozen toes, had combined to wrap me in an overdose of warmth. I sat up, listening to the dark stillness of the country and the patter of drizzle on the roof.

As I struggled to recall the tumble of dreams, I remembered how deeply involved I had become in the shaping of this book, and the memories it had awakened. I recalled clearly a number of items I had raised for discussion with you. I had talked about my horror at dissecting a frog, which surprisingly was much worse than dissecting a dead person. I spoke of my friend Anna and how badly I'd felt about her flunking out. I'd mentioned the competitive stress of students, for which I'd jokingly suggested the importation of soothing Eastern monks. I had talked about the loss of friendship as a result of demanding studies. There was no doubt that all these concerns had surfaced during my nightmare.

I would like to share the dream with you, even though it is very personal, since I believe that it demonstrates how complex human motivation and reaction can be when one is deciding to study medicine. It may also show how inaccessible the understanding of this can be to us. I run a slight risk of frightening you again, but that is the chance I am taking. Let's see what you can make out of the dreams.

I. I was looking through a book, divided into chapters, which nevertheless was a real experience, happening to me even as I watched it. Each chapter enacted an episode of human torture, in which large groups of men were being massacred and made to suffer physically, in the most terrible way imaginable. Although much of this was shrouded in mist, I could catch glimpses of anguished faces, bloodied and mutilated bodies, and hear pleas for mercy. Many of these men appeared to be strapped to tables (like operating or dissecting tables?), and were rendered quite powerless to offer any self-protection. They were "painted" in lavenders and bluish grays, the kinds of colors Renaissance artists would use to portray dead or dying saints. As I passed through and experienced chapter after chapter, my horror and terror mounted.

II. I met a friend who owned a shop next door to

my apartment house in the old neighborhood in Brooklyn Heights. He passed me on the elevator without speaking, and I felt very left behind and "rejected."

III. Two lovely young women in a room were about to be executed by a third, vengeful woman. The first young woman pleaded for her life. She was wearing a two-piece, bright-red satin costume, much like those worn in the South American movie extravaganzas of Bob Hope and Dorothy Lamour. As the "executioner" moved in to kill, I noticed that she intended to do it by stomping the high stiletto heel of her shoe into the young woman's groin, as if that sudden pressure had the power to cause very severe pain and suffering, followed by death. I shuddered, waiting for the lethal shoe to fall. Then, suddenly, miraculously, the woman relented and let the victim run away to safety. My relief was short-lived, however, for even as she ran away, the woman turned to kill the *other* young woman in the room. I had the feeling it might be me.

IV. There was another episode in the "book" mentioned earlier. It told the "story" of an East Indian man of prominence, perhaps a politician-statesman, who was killed by an assassin who had a book containing a bomb delivered to the victim. Opening the door to an innocent-looking person bearing a book-bomb, the man was blown away. My dream also showed a home-movie film of the victim, taken a few days before the event, in which

he looked very much alive and human, thus
increasing the poignancy of the tragic event.
He was completely bald.

That was the end of the dreams. I know that I could spend
hours, over a long period of time, trying to understand the meaning of this very complex and rich piece of nocturnal imagination.
I probably will do it, too. But not now. What I would like to do
now is to point out some things that can be learned quickly,
although, unfortunately, a bit superficially.

The men being destroyed while strapped to dissecting tables
possibly represent in exaggerated and distorted form *all* the
students, animals, and physicians who have had to sacrifice and
suffer in fulfillment of the need of a demanding profession. There
is no doubt in my mind that a vestigial part of me *does* equate
medicine with torture and suffering, in which healers and victims,
physicians and patients, are all wrapped up in some undifferenti-
ated, wrenching process that involves inflicting pain as much as
effecting its relief. Facing and confronting this is so unpleasant,
it is no wonder that we all try to avoid thinking about it. Some
people are fortunate enough to have nightmares on occasion.
Others push it down even further and lock it totally away. A rare
few have the opportunity to be able to talk about it and discuss
it with their teachers and friends, who, I hope, are more attuned
and able to deal with it than people were when I was a student!

The dream fragment in which my friend walked past me in the
elevator reflects a small piece of "real life." The last time I saw
this man, I chewed him out for neglecting me after I'd moved
away. I was annoyed with him for not reaching out more to maintain our friendship, and I did not realize until just this moment
that perhaps I have been feeling guilty, too, for having contributed
to this state of affairs. After all, it takes two to make a friendship,
doesn't it? I'm sure my discussion about the loss of friends brought
all of this to eruption during the night. I am definitely going to
call him up and apologize.

Let me say a word about the woman in the two-piece sarong, for undoubtedly she represented Anna. I believe it was *I* who was the potential woman killer in this dream! I "saved" Anna from "death" at the last moment by "permitting" her to flunk out. I was not so merciful to myself. The stiletto heel might as well have been a fatal knife. It would pain me very much to think that I really think of medicine as "death," and "flunking out" as an escape into life. Although I realize that a part of me does symbolically react this way, it is not the whole story. Although many old memories have been awakened by my undertaking this book, I have not lost sight of the fact that seeking to understand the nature of life, and learning how to preserve it, is the most enriching and rewarding professional life a human being can have. Physicians flirt with death all the time. They fight it, they endure, they accept it, they come to terms with it or they don't. But life and death do permeate their unconscious minds, and some spillover can take place.

I believe that the man who was "blown up" by the "bookbomb," a man who represented tranquility and self-satisfaction, may actually have been a reference to you, my reader. As already expressed, I think a part of me was concerned that my book would indeed come to you as a bomb in the mail, a bomb that might blow you right out of the profession, even as it was delivered by a meek and seemingly inoffensive delivery person (me). Somehow, I got this man jumbled up with the bald-headed monk, who was supposed to be teaching all of us to slow down and brake our frantic racing through life.

Confusing but enlightening nightmares are occasionally the lot of medical students who are reacting to the exploding world in which they live. Even seasoned physicians may awaken in the middle of the night, dreaming for the hundredth time that they have flunked an exam and will have to repeat the year in school! Spouses can do little more than grumble good-naturedly when their sleep is disturbed over this. On this occasion, there is no one for me to disturb but the woodchuck who has gotten into the basement through a hole under the sill, and thinks he owns the place. Unless I have disturbed *you*!

Never mind! The sun is coming up, and it is going to be a glorious day. I will probably be tempted to hit the lake after all these days of rain. Why don't *you* take a break, too, and have some fun? After all, doctors should know how to compartmentalize their lives!

If any of you should wish to become psychiatrists (if only to help your fellow physicians learn to analyze their dreams), we can surely use you. Fewer than 3 percent of today's graduates elect this specialty and it is a great loss to humanity. Think about that!

5.
More
Grubby
Practices

THE DEVELOPMENT OF ADMINISTRATIVE SKILLS

Now that I've had breakfast and a swim, let's resume our discussion of the strategies and forces needed for survival in medical training.

When the director of the residency program in which I used to work announced one day that she had arranged for a time-management seminar for the professional staff, I had difficulty keeping a straight face. As far as the doctors were concerned, it was like sending Sally Rand to Gypsy Rose Lee to teach her how to strip. Good grief! How did that woman think they all got through medical school? If they hadn't learned how to exploit every second of their working lives for maximum efficiency by then, they were a pretty hopeless bunch!

Nevertheless, it did make me realize that time, resource, and personnel management starts for doctors in undergraduate days and goes on until they are planning which golf course in Florida will best suit their retirement needs. You're either an organizer by nature (and most doctors are) or you aren't, but there are skills that anyone can learn. These include learning how to evaluate and use your resources, how to make do with what you have, and how to make sure you get what you need when you need it. Every pre-med I know could benefit from a management course that teaches the principles of measuring efficiency and effectiveness, how to set reasonable goals and objectives for study, how to do a "needs assessment," how to set up some simple systems designs and programs for yourself, and how to monitor your own performance, among other things. You need to be able to do this on a more sophisticated level than apportioning one chapter per hour, from 8:00 P.M. to 2:00 A.M., and again from 6:00 A.M. to 8:00 A.M., only to discover that the test is covering *nine* chapters! Listen to Aunt Naomi and get your act together.

Pre-meds need to learn how to establish "end-points," as they're called in the management business. That means simply knowing where to stop. No matter how hard you study, sooner or later you will meet a situation where you are called upon to produce before you have finished assimilating your material. Your aplomb under these trying circumstances will stand you in good stead when you get out into the "real world" and find that you are functioning on pure, unadulterated aplomb for hours at a time!

Once you've decided to study medicine, *time* becomes both your friend and your enemy. If you don't believe me, ask your doctor advisers. Ask them what they crave the most, ask them what they have the least to spare, ask them what they'd swap their Maseratis for, and they'll all say, *"Time!"* This is said even by those who have trained themselves down to four hours of sleep a night, and are just about walking around with in-dwelling catheters in their bladders to save themselves unnecessary trips to the john.

Nor is this lack of time *value free*. Implicit in the confrontation with the clock is that there might have been more of this precious substance if they had only been better at managing, preserving, spending, or organizing it. Whenever a doctor confesses to running out of time, it is as much an admission of *guilt* as an announcement that he or she has built a successful practice and/or academic career that eats it all up. No doubt about it! If doctors could bottle and sell time, buy it on the stock exchange, or bury it until such time as it would have appreciated x number of dollars a minute, they would surely do so.

Making time your servant is imperative. Why not get some good books on the subject? I suggest *How to Get Control of Your Time and Your Life* by Alan Lakein.

While you're managing your time and resources, remember to apportion your energy. It takes plenty of raw stamina and a good healthy constitution for human animals to keep going under pressure. Think of your body as a temple, and keep it swept, mopped, and weeded. Don't beat yourself around like an old shoe. Don't chintz on your sleep if you don't have to. Don't waste yourself on activities that contribute nothing to the cause of educating, relaxing, or developing you in the broadest sense. Don't go out in the rain without your rubbers. (And don't listen to people who preach.)

THE DISPENSATION WITH RELEVANCE

When I was in school, people were passive about studying what they were told to an extent we'd consider shocking today. We stuffed down raw facts and principles the way some kids eat spinach, knowing that if they make any static, they don't get their Twinkies. I suppose on some primitive level they think that if it tastes so awful, it must be good for them.

Then, around 1965, a movement swept through student circles in this country that questioned many of the time-honored principles of education. (Whenever something is considered "time-honored," you can bet it doesn't have too much else going for it.) One of the issues raised was "relevance," or the revolutionary idea that people shouldn't be asked to learn anything that didn't have some meaning for them, or that could not be proved to demonstrate a concrete connection to their work. This meant, of course, that course content had to be continually evaluated, and thrown out of the curriculum if need be. (You can imagine the ruffled

feathers of those teachers whose material was branded "irrelevant.")
In an era where new knowledge was exploding from every corner,
the movement was as inevitable and necessary as a good dose of
castor oil. We are still feeling the fallout and, by and large, it is to
your advantage. You now have an institutional right to challenge
that was simply not available to us in the old days.

Of course, you have a problem, too. How are you supposed to
know what is relevant and what isn't, when you are at a point in
your training when everything is new and confusing? Aha! Gotcha!
It's the old Catch 22. Half the time you don't know what *is*
relevant, and you're too scared to take a chance and deliberately
not learn it. Well, never mind. It was a great idea. And sometimes
it works.

It is too bad that people aren't allowed to learn in their own
way, as adults who have identified their needs and priorities, and
are simply helped to go out and acquire what they need. But
medical schools and the colleges that "prep" for them are still stuck
in the old stuff-'em-full-of-content routine. I have called this
section *the dispensation with relevance* because sometimes you
just have to give up the struggle to understand why you *need* all
this stuff, and simply take it on faith. Since by definition you are
the kind of person who can't take *anything* on faith, the whole
process may be more than a little hard on you. But the alternative
is worse.

Look at it this way. Isn't it bad enough that you have to memorize the 37 causes of metabolic breakdown, the origins and inser-
tions of 1,482 muscles, and the 349 manifestations of *dementia
praecox* without having to simultaneously torture yourself over
whether or not this nonsense is *important*? That way madness lies.
A good hustler, who really enjoys the blood lust of competition,
will keep his doubts, gripes, grouses, and discontentment under
control. All instincts to book burning, academic revolution, and
curricular foment will be ruthlessly checked, the better to advance
your greater goal of somehow becoming a physician before you
get *dementia praecox* yourself.

But may I suggest keeping detailed notes and observations for later reference? That way you can comfort yourself with the thought that someday you will write the great American doctor novel, based on your personal journal, and that it will forever change the idiocy of the medical education process. By then, of course, you may have mellowed, and will be busy revising your concepts of relevance. I personally have always had trouble reconciling the pursuit of relevance with the pursuit of knowledge. Such sentiments are shared by research scientists, who see analogies in the restrictions based on "pure" or "basic" science versus "applied" science.

It is possible that much of the rebellion on campuses against irrelevance is actually a rebellion against infantilization, a process that envelops undergraduates and medical students alike. Since infantilization is twice as insulting when one is simultaneously given direct responsibility for the management of human life and death, we will discuss it further when we talk more about life in medical school. But be prepared for a lot of this in college. The truth is, they make you learn a lot of dumb stuff. And they treat you as if you were in kindergarten. It's disgusting.

THE NARROWING OF CULTURAL HORIZONS

I suppose one of the appraisals people have to make about themselves when still in high school is whether they are merely bright or truly intellectual in outlook. You have to be clever and cerebral to make it in medical school, but you don't have to be a real intellectual. As a matter of fact, it's rather a handicap.

Intellectuals may become excellent doctors, but they find the training period more agonizing, simply because it is no longer possible to think independently. Putting a real intellectual into medical school is a bit like hitching a Derby runner behind a slow milk wagon. People like this undergo withdrawal symptoms when they can't run out to the latest foreign flick, can't take the time for a well-considered letter to the editor, no longer get to theater, ballet, symphony without feeling that they are betraying mankind by doing it. Such people will be particularly sensitive to the parochial and narrow interests they will perceive in their teachers, and more inclined to disillusionment with the power politics, vested scientific interests, and rigid academic categorizations of the medical curriculum. They will chafe particularly at dogma, grow restless under the thumb of the rote lecturer. Or perhaps they will grow bored with the irrelevancies to which they will be exposed.

But there is hope for them. They should be assured that if they can put up with the confining attitudes, they will rise to the top of the profession. Those who value them will bathe them in honor and affection, and look to them for leadership in all aspects of personal and professional life. *The New England Journal of Medicine* will eagerly accept their writings under the "Sounding Board" (editorial) section of the journal. They will organize "Humanities and Medicine" courses at their alma maters, which the social workers will attend. They will be sought after as speakers on educational occasions, where others of the profession may even listen to them. And most important, they will be working in a field offering them unlimited possibilities to learn, grow, and contribute when the next twelve years are over. So if you have been a gifted child, functioning in a "normal" school, you will have had a taste of what it means to be a creative and unusual person in a traditional learning situation. That's what you will find in your chosen field. Use your ingenuity and good humor to modify or soften the system as much as you can. If *you* don't do it, who will?

By the way, even folks who make no pretensions of loving learning for its own sake will feel the pinch in undergraduate and medical school. Bookstores, libraries, concert halls, museums, convention halls, planetariums, and all other repositories of human civilization wouldn't last long if all the world were populated by doctors.

I have always found it an amazing paradox that physicians who master a universe of material are often considered dull clods by people who have to put up with their behavior at parties. It is hard to convince laypeople that they should have sincere respect for a profession so compelling it could make social boors of its practitioners. Doctors do voluntarily renounce much of the world's culture and civilization to pursue their lives' work. No value judgment there. Just a statement of fact. Know it before you start. If you are determined not to lose the glories of our civilization, think twice. And if you choose medicine still, plan your specialty wisely. A special welcome to you!

SENSORY DEPRIVATION AND TEMPORARY REALITY LOSS

I made reference earlier to how miserable it can be for students when the sun shines, the birds tweet, and the wind rustles seductively in the ears. Students locked up in their cages during exam week can suffer plenty, particularly if they are fond of Elizabethan poetry that never lets anyone forget that life is fleeting, youth ephemeral, April the cruelest month, and blossoms quick to wilt.

> Gather ye rosebuds while ye may,
>   Old time is still a-flying,
> And this same flower that blooms today,
>   Tomorrow may be dying.

I mention this because, in some foolish way, long-term students *do* get gypped out of many real, sensory pleasures accruing to others merely by virtue of their youth, good spirits, and relative freedom from worries.

Examples? For some people, being cooped up during the first tentative days of spring is especially hard. There are some moments when you feel like an animal pacing in a room, simply screaming to be let out to feel the wind on your face. On such days, you simply light out, and work as hard as possible to make up for it another time when temptation isn't such a problem. Of course, that isn't always possible.

Like students in many professional schools, students of medicine suffer from lack of sleep. They get torn from their beds on cold winter mornings, when the enveloping warmth of their blankets protects like a mommy's arms. They are prevented from crawling back in at night by mountains of books, notes, slides, and a week's worth of dirty clothes. Sleep is something most people can usually take for granted. Who would think that for some it would be as forbidden as an ice-cream sundae, a trip to Cuba, or a weekend with some fantasy sex object.

Doctors in training probably don't get enough cuddling. If it were possible to let people take "snuggling" instead of "phys-ed," they'd probably all turn out for the better. This deprivation is part of being a college student who is often far from home, without too much privacy, autonomy, or good snuggling partners. But it's a loss. Bring your old teddy with you just in case.

At this point, it is important to say something about sex, although the subject has been hashed into the ground by just about everybody with a typewriter and some morbid interest in the manipulation of human needs. Actually, it is really nobody's business but that of the individual student, and few of us are in a position to offer meaningful assistance to people who have to work out their adult dilemmas by themselves. Although I'm reluctant to write about it at all, I don't want to cop out. If there's help I can add, these are my thoughts.

In an age where most people feel no barriers to sexual experiences of many kinds, and therefore indulge themselves almost at whim, the pre-medical and medical student may be forgiven for thinking in his or her more paranoid moments that this sensory pleasure, too, has been snatched away by an all-consuming and vengeful god of medicine. In a sense it may be true that informal and casual sex is another victim of the demands of being a doctor. Only you can make the judgment of how great this loss would be to you, if at all.

The reality is that students without spouse-type people to love usually don't have too much time or energy to find others, or to cultivate them when they do. (Life might be easier for students if someone could assign them a spouse along with their gym lockers and lab equipment.) Even when the atmosphere is full of eligible sex objects, it is often stressful for student doctors to gather their rosebuds, an occupation that their parents, teachers, and hang-ups appear to view as having no redeeming intellectual value whatsoever. Gathering rosebuds also fails to sit well with those of the opposite sex, particularly women, who get the feeling that they are being rushed, used, and exploited in the mad, one-night-a-week pursuit of horticulture.

Nevertheless, many students have no problems whatsoever in finding companions and having great fun. Others have their ups and downs. Also, there are some students who choose to temporarily give up the unequal struggle to satisfy sensory needs at the expense of human feelings, and postpone it for a later day, substituting the other satisfactions they feel more appropriate to their position. That makes a certain sense to me. Contrary to popular belief, human beings can grow and develop nicely without their genitals being massaged on a regular basis. Sex was never a function mandated by the vital centers of the human organism, like circulation, respiration, and eructation following an Italian meal. Those who spend their early student years giving priorities to other items on their agenda, either from principle or realistic necessity, will be happy to discover that the Elizabethans were unduly influenced by their short expected life span of thirty-five. People live twice as long today, and have discovered the joys of geriatric sex. Knowing that it's there and it isn't going to go away for a long time should be a help when the caged sexual animal starts to pace and wants to be let out. Roses may slip through your fingers, but there's a whole garden out there—and to every flower its season.

Without necessary precautions, long-term students may find themselves foregoing the pleasures of a healthy body. They tend to sit around in libraries and labs like hippopotamuses, developing large posteriors, flabby thighs, and little curly tails. They don't take time for exercise, become claudicated and winded before their time, and never get to feel the sense of well-being that comes from a sleek, tuned-up body functioning like a well-oiled machine. It is an awesome warning of what is to come in the future. My eight-year-old BMW is in better shape than I am. Since there's no need to sound like an editorial exhortation on the dust cover of a diet or exercise manual, I'll rein in the gloom-and-doom pronouncements. Instead, I'll just put you on notice that studying medicine can be damaging to your health. The surgeon-general should be required to have all medical schools put warning notices to that effect on the covers of their academic bulletins.

More startling to me than the deprivation of sensory pleasures is the student's temporary loss of reality, and resultant suspension in a fixed world of study. It's not easy to explain what I mean. Let me give you an example. When I was working at my first position following residency, I turned on the TV one day and found a rather funny situation comedy that starred Lucille Ball and Desi Arnaz. It was about a very appealing, highly manipulative, sex-stereotyped, redheaded woman, the wife of a bandleader who played corny South American music and had a heavy accent. As I let the series come into my home daily at the dinner hour (anything to avoid the news), I became impressed with the comic genius of the heroine. Noting the long skirts and antique autos, I figured that it must be a replay of some older series, like Sid Caesar or Red Skelton. I told a friend that I'd stumbled on something called *I Love Lucy*, and discovered for the first time that I was finally being exposed to a program that had been the rage of America years before. I'd missed it completely. I'd been studying.

Students can get caught in a real time warp, as they miss seminal events in the world, magazines, books, and movies, etc. I personally missed the entire Korean war—also, many fads, whole wardrobes of the latest fashions, and key obituaries, discovering years later which persons of note had died during my tenure as a student.

I also recall one day when not one student doctor showed up for the dermatology clinic at the Philadelphia General Hospital. I was there all alone to care for forty-three walking skin diseases. The reason? The first moon shot was taking place, and the whole world stayed home to watch it on television. Everyone, that is, except forty-three people with an itch, and one medical student who had an unusually bad case of time warp.

As holidays go by unobserved, as white sales pass unnoticed, as specials like *Roots* are bypassed, as human rituals like sleeping, playing soccer, and buying a new razor go unremembered, medical students and pre-meds tend to develop transient feelings of unreality. The only consolation one can offer is to note that much that goes on in the world is worth skipping anyway, and some pleasures, like *I Love Lucy*, come back again and again.

THE TRANSIENCE OF EXULTATION

I don't know where you could have gotten this idea, but you may have the impression that a student doctor's life is a stressful one. True. But that is not to say it is devoid of its moments of sheer exaltation.

Consider the following. Word has it that the qualitative analysis exam is going to be a short-answer, multiple-choice quiz that hits and runs all over the element chart. But *your* hunch says that the instructor may ask you to write an essay about one or more of his favorite elements, such as silver or gold. So, you make it your business to be prepared. As a hustler, you know that you could be squandering precious knowledge-acquisition time, and that the outcome will either leave you dripping with the blood lust of competition, or suffering a severe case of survivor guilt. But this time you really want to be creative about your studying, so you go for broke on several selected elements. Sure enough, the exam is a one-question quiz, stating simply, "Write everything you know about either (gold) or (silver)." You do. And you walk out of the room looking like the cat that swallowed the half and half. You "creamed" the course, you'll get a certain A, and the most delicious case of survivor guilt ever to be drowned in an evening of beer drinking.

There are no words to describe the euphoria occasioned by such a coup! No other human being could possibly understand the surge of adrenalin that pounds through your major vessels, your ears, your eyeballs, and your unmassaged reproductive organs. But just as quickly, it goes! The next morning the grind starts all over again.

Experience makes us reluctantly conclude that exultation is transient. It can't be stored up. Get used to this, too. The Talmud put it nicely, *Gam zeh ya-avor* (This, too, shall pass). Wonderful moments are like splashes of cold water thrown on your face to revive you for another round with the champion who's using you for a punching bag. But they're wonderful. Enjoy every second— even when you can count them on the fingers of one hand.

THE ROLLER-COASTER EGO

You should know about the quadrennial cycle that determines the way student doctors feel about themselves. It's all been programmed into them. It starts in college when a freshman is on the first anticipatory flush of the chosen career. It lasts only until the student opens the books and realizes that he or she is but a lowly academic *worm*. It's a steady climb up the status tree until graduation, when, with luck, the whole process starts all over again.

The medical student is now a miserable freshman worm reincarnated. Although it's the second time during this roller-coaster career, it won't be the last. In four more years, the medical-school senior will become a miserable *intern*, and have to climb through four years of postgraduate training.

Wouldn't you think that a doctor finishing a long residency in a hospital would be capable enough to get out and start a practice with the respect of the community? Of course! Only now that doctor is a miserable "junior attending" at the local sawbones factory, and has to work back up through the ranks to obtain privileges, patients, and some measure of control over the conditions of his or her practice. It takes at least fifteen years out of high school before a doctor can look in the mirror and say without a shadow of a doubt, "I have arrived. I am no longer a miserable worm!" By then, the ego has been on so many ups and downs, it's no wonder stabilization seems a lifelong task. So, be prepared for feeling like the king of the jungle one minute, and the mouse that squeaked the next. It's all part of the game.

INTEGRATING YOURSELF

The pre-medical years are years in which students spend a lot of time taking themselves apart and putting themselves back together again. That's understandable when we consider that we have been talking about so many things that really have nothing to do with mastery of a body of didactic knowlege, but deal instead with self-knowledge and accommodation to a remarkably demanding and unspontaneous system of education. On some level, potential medical students know this. So do those who have considered the field and rejected it because "it's too hard." I have written this book because I would like people to know where they are heading—not to encourage them unduly, or keep them out unnecessarily, but just to enable them to make an informed decision. And the most important thing they have to consider in saying yes or no is that they won't be the same persons coming out that they were when they went in. Never mind the hard work. They will have to take themselves apart and put themselves back together again.

Let me run down some of the challenges that will be arising before an acceptance even arrives! Students will have to be hustlers: aggressive, forthright, take-charge, self-determining people. Some of this can be learned, some must be instinct. Not all of it is good; in fact, a good bit can be contaminating and deleterious to the personality. Maybe someday admissions committees will wise up and stop setting up academic conditions that force students into unhealthy roles and attitudes. But utopia isn't here yet, and you haven't time to wait. Can you handle it, and integrate whatever competitive instincts you may need into your gentle personality?

Students have to be tenacious, refusing to give up no matter how bleak things may seem. They may have to do this without enough emotional support, and despite the counsel of well-meaning friends. They will have to endure much loneliness, particularly as they become survivors of preordained attrition in the ranks. They will have to postpone many pleasures, and give up some entirely for a while, substituting some rather terrifying experiences. They will have to learn to work together with one another, even as they are in competition with each other.

They may have to revise their concepts of right and wrong, and deal with a succession of values in conflict. They will have to learn to be superorganizers, individuals who maintain control over their time and actions. They will have to sift a lot of wheat from a lot of chaff, and deal with the trauma of not knowing which is which, while still recognizing that errors could be fatal. They will have to give up much that was good and beautiful in their lives, and recognize that never again will there be time to indulge these things as they should be. They will have to deal with triumph that is fleeting, and despair that can haunt for hours and days on end. Most important, they will inevitably face self-doubt and the fear of failure, and will have to learn to live with it the way the handicapped survive with their own more tangible impediments. They will have to learn to like themselves even when they hate themselves, and discipline themselves even when they most cry out to break away free. They will have to develop a realistic way of appraising their weaknesses and accomplishments, for the enforcements and reinforcements of the outside world may be inappropriate, untimely, or excessive in their presence or absence. They will have to maintain a handle on what they are truly doing for themselves, what they are doing for others, and, if need be, accept the right things for the wrong reasons, and the wrong things for the right reasons.

And when they're all done, they have to put it all together in a neat little package that hopes to put an M.D. after its name. They'll have to integrate a hundred processes that are going on concurrently, and none of which seem to make any sense until much later, if at all. If they succeed, no one will know, and if they fail, they will never let themselves forget it. The end of the story will not be written for many years. The beginning is now.

6.
Roulette

A certain expectant electricity charges the air when fall arrives in the senior year. The ritual of medical-school applications takes precedence for the first time over the religion of pure study. Some students will apply to forty or fifty schools, proof of their eagerness, insecurity, and poor judgment; others will apply to only one or two, testifying equally well to their "cool" but even worse judgment. Most will contact a reasonable number, which is smart, because schools charge for evaluating their applicants and these fees have a way of adding up.

The fall is a season of reckoning. It is a prolonged "moment of truth." It is a time of dressing up in toreador costume in the hope that somewhere out there in that great academic bull ring there's a big fat bovine with your name on it. For some students, application is only a necessary technicality. They know that they have been looked on with favor by one or more schools, and the anxiety is only token. Others must sweat it out until the bitter end. The months that intervene between the submission of applications and the welcome letter of acceptance can drag on like Chinese water torture. It is a grim reality that repeated and unrelieved rejection slips will be the fate of many solid hustlers.

Since I began this first section of the book with my own experience, I will end it the same way. Those who have been in the ring will recognize that the story is not all that remarkable. Others, who have yet to win their ears, may find it useful. Olé!

It began to occur to me that I might not get into medical school in October of that final year of college. It was the first time I had been able to admit such a possibility to myself, although the warning indicators had been around in abundance since that infamous train ride from Brooklyn back to Delaware several years before.

It was true that I had gotten "straight A's" in all my courses in advanced literature, writing, history, language, and other allied subjects. But it was also true that I had barely squeaked by in biology, math, physics, and chemistry. I had taken the fewest possible science courses, figuring that most would be repeated in medical school (as indeed they were, to the infinite boredom of my more traditional classmates). But those that I *did* take had given me trouble.

By the time applications were to be mailed away, I'd had ample time to reflect on my horrendous grades, my anxieties and terrors when confronted for the first time in my life with the realities of nature and laboratory science, and my humble position with regard to the other competitors for my place in the freshman class. It suddenly seemed to matter little that I had been transformed from a sheltered, naive, dreamy-eyed, bright, articulate young person into a competitive, blood-lusting hustler; a tenacious survivor into the semifinals; a tough, independent, battle-scarred and very senior pre-medical candidate. Momentarily forgotten were all the positive, perhaps exceptional attributes that other people had recognized, attributes that were as necessary to the development of a good physician as a natural aptitude for the scientific method. The only thing I was aware of was that I was inadequate, presumptuous in my dreams, out of my depth, and pursuing some mad folly.

Given the circumstances, this was not such an inaccurate appraisal of myself. But what I have since learned is that it is a fairly characteristic feeling of almost *all* pre-meds! There is something about the current educational process that feeds self-doubt, feelings of personal inadequacy, and expectations of failure—and by now you are gaining some understanding of what they are. I hope it will not always be that way. One of my hopes for the future is to edit a book of essays written by successful physicians of all ages, specialties, and medical schools, describing their personal odysseys through the pre-medical and medical student world, and discussing how they coped, matured, and/or were scarred by their experiences. Perhaps it might help those yet to come.

The wait through the winter months was by no means a totally passive one. By now the "mutual support" network was in full operation, as former competitors compared notes. It became rapidly apparent that I had made the classic mistake (but one perfectly consistent with my delusions of grandeur) of applying primarily to the top-flight schools. Although all American medical schools are now supposed to be grade A, there is no secret to the fact that some are more prestigious than others. I should have expected my rejections from Penn, Columbia, New York University, and others of that ilk. I cursed the misguided relation who had advised me to apply to them, obviously failing to consider that my generation was going to have a harder time getting into medical school than had his.

Milton called me one day in February. "Now look," he said, "my school wanted to reject you outright. But I worked on the admissions committee and succeeded in having them pull your name from the bottom of the barrel. They'll give you an interview. But no promises!" It turned out to be a good thing that no promises were made, for his school, too, rejected me, after a cursory interview with a gray little man in a gray suit who asked me some gray questions and then informed me that he considered me to be "impelled" rather than "motivated." He thought I would be a poor candidate to stick it out.

As my wait stretched out into March, then April, I began to panic. My grade point index to date was an abysmal 2.83! I had applied to eight schools, and had received seven rejections in as many months. All around me classmates were being accepted, and there I sat. My hopes were pinned on the final school remaining.

I mentioned earlier that stress can make highly ethical people behave in ways that seem inconsistent with their usual philosophy of life. As all the doors slammed in my face, I succumbed to temptation. I picked up the phone and called one of my uncles, a prominent hospital administrator and physician who had pioneered a number of highly innovative social movements in medicine. "Uncle," I wailed, "I am beside myself. Would you please call the dean at the Woman's Medical College of Pennsylvania and ask her to consider my application? I am not asking for any favors, only an opportunity to come and plead my case. I *know* I can do the work, if she will just give me a chance." I was close to tears. I guess it was probably the single most humiliating thing I ever had to do. To this day, the ethical lapse still abrades me. I am bothered by the thought that I used an asset not available to the thousands of other students who wanted in as badly as I did—an influential relative.

However, I could have spared myself the *mea culpa*'s. He would have none of it. His answer, as I recall it, was, "I am sorry. If you can't get in without me, you are not going to get in *because* of me!" I would have to go the final round alone. I remember being hurt and angry. It had been so hard for me to call. And to have all the humiliation, all the guilt, and none of the worldly rewards! This reaction was reinforced by all those to whom I confided the story. ("What a terrible thing to do, not to help someone in need!") To this day, when I tell people that there are still persons of high moral rectitude in the profession, their reaction is unappreciative derision. I confess to being unsure how I feel about it now myself. And yet, as things turned out, I lived to be delighted that he'd turned me down.

By forcing me to stand or fall on my own, he aborted at least some of the feelings of guilt over the request. He reinforced my gut reaction that although it may have been humanly right, it was morally wrong. He released me from a lifetime of obligation to him, for there was no way I could ever have repaid him. Most important, he freed me from the haunting feeling that "I never made it on my own." This is something that more and more people torture themselves with nowadays, particularly women and minorities. Most of the time, they more than deserve what they were given.

I immediately buried the unpleasant incident. And I waited as the weeks dragged into May. One day, about four weeks before graduation, I realized that I was going to have to make alternate arrangements for the coming September. Like many other students who had refused to accept the possibility of defeat until very late, I was going to have to scramble for a job or a place in graduate school. I traveled into town for a visit to the psychiatrist who had given me so much encouragement over two and one-half years before. I cried for over an hour. It was a catharsis of no mean proportions. I guess I had to go through it before I could even begin to plan a future. It was probably the supreme act of acceptance for me, and he was very kind to let me mess up his hours while I used his office for my ordeal.

"Now," he said, "where are you going to go from here?" Thoroughly cleansed by my tears, I surprised myself and made an instantaneous decision. I dried my eyes and said, "I am going to go to graduate school at the University of Pennsylvania, for a master's degree in biology. I will reapply after one year, or two years, if need be. Perhaps they will take me if I prove that I can handle the work at that level." And I left, determined not to give up, ready for the next round, and feeling comforted in some strange way that my fight was not yet over. It was a stupid decision, of course. Although one or two years of graduate school can help a potential candidate, it sometimes constitutes good years thrown after bad, and the longer one hangs in, the more diminished the ultimate chance of acceptance. For me, there was no other choice. Even as I accepted failure, I had to continue to deny it for a while.

Because of the unusual lateness of the hour, I stopped at a phone booth to let my parents know that I'd be late for dinner. (I lived at home during my last semester to save some money.) To my great surprise, my father answered the phone. "We expected you hours ago," he said impatiently. Hoping that the excessive nasal quality of my voice wouldn't betray me, I apologized. "Look here," he continued, "there's a letter for you."

Since this was the first time in twenty years that he had bothered to announce the existence of a mere letter, and since his voice held an edge of suppressed excitement. I felt the adrenalin start to pour through my visceral arterioles.

"From whom?"

"The Woman's Medical College of Pennsylvania."

"Open it!"

"I did!"

At this point I paused. My father, as full of moral rectitude as his brother, had never in his life opened an envelope addressed to another human being. I was overwhelmed that he had violated his own code in deference to the need to help me with the con- . tents of that final envelope. He must have known that he would be needed to comfort or celebrate with me.

"What did it say?"

His voice was trembling with excitement. *"It says that you have been accepted as a member of the incoming freshman class! Congratulations, my daughter!"*

I had no tears left. I was terribly tired. But I was happy. And I was grimly pleased, even in my moment of triumph, that I had done it without anyone's intervention.

I am a sentimental fool. I sometimes save letters that have a special meaning for me. For those of you who have never seen a real, live acceptance letter from a real, live medical school, I am pleased to reproduce it for you here in its entirety.

May 19

Miss Naomi Bluestone
401 West 34th Street
Wilmington, Delaware

Dear Miss Bluestone:
    Quite unexpectedly there has been a withdrawal

of one of the accepted students for this coming September. Consequently, the Admissions Committee have recommended you for the class in her place.

It will be necessary for you to take care of the following: filing of the enclosed health forms within two weeks as well as a chest X-ray 14 x 17 inches (paper film not acceptable) sent to the Student Health Department.

One final college transcript and one of your high school are sent from my office to the Pennsylvania State Department of Public Instruction for the issuance of your Pre-Professional certificate. Will you request your high school to send transcripts in duplicate and your college transcripts in duplicate at the end of the year in June.

It is also my understanding that you will meet the requirement of Quantitative Analysis this coming summer in summer school.

College and medical schools generally are finding a tuition increase necessary. The Board of Corporators on April 25, 1958, authorized an increase in tuition of $100.00 making a yearly total of $1,000.00.

To insure your place in the class, the enclosed letter is to be signed and returned with the deposit of $50.00 by June 2, 1958.

Sincerely yours,

M. Elizabeth Huston
Administrative Assistant

I have often thought how much pain I could have spared myself had I decided to postpone my nervous breakdown by just one more day. As it was, I felt like a fool groping in my pocket for another dime to call back the man I'd just left to say, "I've been accepted after all." But true medical masochist that I am, I cannot honestly say in retrospect that I am sorry. I think it was important for me to go through the agony of believing and trying to accept the fact of my ultimate rejection. It is very important, in my opinion, for a physician to have experienced a searing failure at least once in his or her life, for without it there is no true maturity, no empathy for others who are failing, and no self-pity or understanding when therapeutic efforts do not succeed.

To say that I was grateful to the Woman's Medical College for accepting me is to issue the understatement of the year. I had pinned high hopes in Philadelphia, for this had been the only school to even give me an interview (with the exception of the employers of the gray man in Brooklyn who had issued moral pronouncements on my character in what I would now consider to be an unethical and intrusive way). They had also made the interview, by tradition a grim initiation rite, an educational and supporting experience.

To those of you worrying about admissions interviews, let me digress an instant and tell you about this particular one. I had gone to it expecting the cursory brushoff I'd had in Brooklyn at the more traditional school. For that reason, I had not bothered to empty my bladder before arriving, a fatal mistake, and I was too overawed and embarrassed to be able to ask for relief during the four ensuing hours. I was met by each of four or five women in a variety of clinical and pre-clinical specialties, all of whom expressed sincere interest in me and my plans for the future. Giving me a tour of the school and taking me to lunch, they questioned me and answered questions, impressing me as warm, caring, unusual human beings.

Yes, it's true that they asked me questions that today would be considered sexist and in violation of my rights to privacy and the lack of self-incrimination. They wanted to know what I would do if I married a man who didn't approve of women doctors, and how I planned to manage a romper room full of kids. But they were well-intentioned, utterly practical, and clearly motivated by the desire to help rather than exclude. I felt no antipathy to answering as honestly as possible. To be truthful, it was the first time I'd really *confronted* the issue of dual role conflict. (It was not surprising in those days, but it *is* surprising now how many people still do not give enough consideration to how they will manage these life situations until they are into them!)

The ladies in Philadelphia made me very happy by telling me that they would have to be guaranteed payment for four years before they could accept me, since they didn't want any students dropping out and sacrificing precious places in the class for mere want of funds. I remember being thrilled that they thought enough of me *even to raise the issue.* I, on the other hand, had progressed no further in my reality planning than the statement I'd once made to Milton, naively boasting about having saved enough money for the first year. (That night, immediate arrangements were made for a guaranteed loan, to assure those nice people that there would be no impediments other than the usual to their acceptance of me.)

When the interview was terminated late in the afternoon, I was excited and hopeful (and in such pain and distress from my overflowing urinary reservoir that I thought I would die). If any of these women are indeed still members of the admissions committee of the college, now known as the Medical College of Pennsylvania, I do hope they will ask as pertinent questions about their candidate's fluid-excretory status as they do about their home lives and fiscal solvency.

Pre-medical students may be forgiven for being obsessed with the admission process. They see it as the culmination of the entire educational experience since high school, the "Grand Prix" of all they have learned.

They have special anxieties about the admissions interview itself. They besiege their elders and betters with all manner of concrete questions about how to comport themselves. "What shall I wear?" "Shall I let them know that my wife is expecting twins?" "Is it appropriate for me to tell a joke?" "Am I supposed to be talkative (assertive, outgoing, extroverted, collegial, etc.), or should I be more silent (passive, retiring, introverted, abject etc.)?" "What if they ask me (fill in the blank)?"

If it weren't so pathetic, I'd be inclined to laugh. The best advice I think anyone can give is "yes." Yes, dress appropriately (and if you don't know what that is by now, nothing is going to help). Yes, be whatever you are. Yes, listen to your interviewer; yes, be responsive; and yes, use your instincts about the whole business. Every interview is its own non-replicatable experience. Yes, enjoy it. And if you don't know what else to say, smile and say yes. By and large, medical schools like people who say yes.

People who have weathered their interviews, which often turn out to be surprisingly informal and fun, and possess an acceptance at a school of their choice (or any school, for that matter—how choosy can you get?) are really crossing over a certain kind of Jordan. Henceforth they will know that they have been chosen, that there is an investment in maintaining them through their training, and that they are now serious apprentices for a serious profession. If at all possible, they should spend their last summer assiduously wasting their time, having fun, shirking responsibilities, accomplishing nothing, sleeping late, retiring not at all, and in general behaving like medieval European university students. They should be the bane of storekeepers, the despair of their parents, and a hideous example for all who come after them. They should be held up as loathsome representatives of what the future of medicine is coming to. ("*This* wants to be a doctor?") And they should pay no heed to the morrow, for it will come soon enough.

Getting
Finished:
Medical
School

7.
Books,
Bones, and
Boredom
(The Pre-Clinical Years)

There are 125 medical schools in this country, and in most of them a student's first responsibility is to take apart a dead human being. This unnerving assignment has to be undertaken just when he or she is settling into a new apartment in a strange town, racing over to the bookstore to pick up the explanatory texts, and trying to find out where the cafeteria is. If you think that this initiation could have been devised by the barbarians, who believed in trial by fire, the flotation of witches, the survival of the fittest, and puberty rites oriented toward wild animals, most civilized pedagogues would probably agree with you.

Horrified by their own remembrances of dissections past, they point out that a formalin-pickled patient sets a bad emotional cast for further clinical studies. The cadaver, after all, is the very embodiment of death, the archenemy. It is at best a most unrewarding creature to deal with when one still doesn't know which parking lot to use. It is as passive as a patient can be, rarely saying, "Ouch, you're hurting me!" or in any other way protesting the invasion of its privacy or its person. Disappearing in small chunks each day under the knives of four students (unless supplies are scarce), the cadaver forces a confrontation with all the terrifying emotions that a raw human being can endure.

The anatomy laboratory is surely the first image that comes to the mind of laypeople and physicians alike when "becoming a doctor" is discussed. A great deal has been written about it, in an attempt to get a handle on the strong feelings it arouses, either anticipatory or retrospective in nature.

One particularly interesting discussion came across my desk recently in the form of an essay by psychiatrist Dr. John Cody. Cody had the unusual experience of going through cadaver dissection *twice*, first as an art student, then five years later as a medical student. He gives a fascinating contrast between the "coping" methods used by artists, who were concerned with the body's artistic form and content, and student physicians, who were obsessed with the minute technical detail that was sure to be on the exam. Giving a graphic description of the realities of the dissecting room, he ventures the opinion that it is indeed very good for students to start out this way, and to have the opportunity to deal with the unspeakable from the very outset. I share his views, instinctively, and wish that more people could read his very fascinating descriptive and analytical essay. It was entitled "The Arts versus Angus Duer," and appeared in a monograph of the Society for Health and Human Values. I commend it to you.

Perhaps someday psychologists and other humane educators will accomplish their goal of letting young physicians begin their studies with an analysis of life and how it functions, rather than death and how it horrifies. Until that time, medical students will continue to deal with the sudden deluge of feelings that can overwhelm on their own.

Many will be able to resurrect from the stark confrontation many positive things. They will feel pride at having encountered and mastered one of the most frightening experiences of medicine. They will feel that they have earned the right in coming years to approach living patients whom they must frequently penetrate as they did the cadaver. They will be imbued with the desire to keep their patients very much alive, so as never to have to confront a cadaver they have known when it was a person who spoke to them. Even in the ordinary process of dissection, they will be teasing out life from death, and the joy of learning will soon overcome the sorrow of death. After all, the human body is such a magnificent creation! At last, all emotion will be buried under the reality needs of passing exams, mastering the work load, and building a base for courses that run concurrently or will soon follow.

Students quickly adjust to gross anatomy. In time, they even grow careless about bringing snacks into the lab, plopping down a bag of brownies beside them as they work. They migrate from the murderous to the mundane in the most remarkable way. (Actually, I got some of my best recipes from one of my cadaver-mates!) Here is an excerpt from a letter that I wrote to my parents after just one week in medical school. Note the rather clear mixture of horror and matter-of-factness, the grisly and the ordinary, served up with bravado and studied carelessness.

Mother . . . I am still up on my work, but probably not for long. We are chipping in for a pencil sharpener and a subscription to the *Inquirer*. . . . I've got a huge box of bones to keep in my room and memorize. It weighs a ton, and includes a grinning skull. Now you'd better turn this over to Daddy or you'll get sick. . . .

Daddy, my cadaver is a six-foot, forty-seven-year-old male Negro, who died four years ago of a pulmonary infarction. I don't know if you had to prepare *your* bodies, but we had to scrape off all the grease coating with a scalpel, shave all the body hair, and wash the body with soap and water. Believe me, I nearly vomited. It's much worse than actual dissection. We are lucky to have such a slender, muscular specimen, but God, does he stink! You should *see* what some of the kids got! . . . In histology we have 175 slides to learn, plus

eight demonstrations per day, and reams of detailed notes already. The whole thing is very boring and I'll be glad when these two years are over.
It's like being back in college again. Dull!

I soon found that it was more important to win the approval of
instructors and to master the material than to indulge in petty pa-
tronization of my mom, who could squash a roach with the tip of
her shoe (which was more than *I* ever could have done). The
romance of anatomy faded, along with the old stories about grave
robbers in Scotland, and the Bowery bums whose bodies could be
purchased (in advance) for fifty cents by prospective medical students in my uncle's day. The push was on to study. Note the hum-
bled quality of another letter sent barely a month later!

. . . Today we had our first real oral exam in six
weeks in gross anatomy lab. We were the last table
the professor visited, having expected him every
day for a week, and nearly dying of apprehension
every day. God, what an ordeal! He tore the two
kids opposite us to shreds for a sloppy, incomplete
dissection, and we died thinking what he was
going to say to *us*, because Seana, my partner,
literally hacked our arm to pieces, for which I
could have killed her. Then he came to us. I was
almost paralyzed. I heard him pick up our arm
and say to the other two women who share our
cadaver, "Now *this* is the way you should have dis-
sected! Do you see how they've cleared out all
their structures?" Well, I was so flabbergasted I
nearly fell under the table, and Seana's mouth
dropped open and she said to him, "You're kidding,"
in a flat statement of disbelief.

Then he got to work on us! The man has a rapier
tongue and a frighteningly powerful intellect. He

headed for the quadrangular space, which I knew *cold*, because I did that particular dissection myself. If you don't remember your anatomy, that's the area where the axillary nerve and the posterior circumflex humeral artery come through. He picked up something and said "Miss Bluestone, what is this?" "That's a nerve, sir," I replied, thinking, "What kind of a goddam stupid question is *that* to ask?" "Exactly," he said, "and which nerve?" "That," I said proudly, forcefully, assuredly, "is the posterior circumflex humeral." There was this terrible silence, before he called on Seana, and I realized what a hideous mistake I had made.

Then I started to laugh. It was so absurd that I should make such an assy error on something I knew so well, when I hadn't learned half the arm! I'm afraid it sounded a little hysterical, because he said, "Miss Bluestone, if you don't stop that childish giggling, I'll give you an A for immaturity." Well, I shut up quick, but I don't remember another question he asked us; I'm absolutely blank. But I guess we passed, because he didn't yell anymore except once. He asked us to demonstrate the *palmaris longus* and Seana picked up this piece of meat off the table and dangled it in the air and said, "Here it is!" He got absolutely apoplectic. Only Seana could destroy a muscle like that and get away with it. She didn't bat an eyelash

We all passed anatomy, just as you will, too. It will not be quite as important a subject for you, as there is much more competitive material to be learned now than there was twenty years ago. But someday you will be able to discuss your initiation with a sense of humor, a matter-of-factness, and some degree of reality.

The two years that begin the medical experience are known

traditionally as the "pre-clinical years," that is, the years before full-time work with patients in the hospital takes over. These freshman and sophomore years are devoted almost exclusively to the laboratory sciences, such as anatomy, physiology, biochemistry, histology, microbiology, genetics, pathology, pharmacology, and the like. Basic science courses, like their predecessors in college, deal in microscopes and instruments of measurement, laboratory equipment and experimental animals, textbooks, notebooks, observations, and records. Personal contact comes primarily from fellow students and laboratory scientists, rather than patients and "clinical" physicians (those who directly treat patients rather than providing support services for those who do).

Most medical students are as uncomfortable with this arrangement as they are beginning their careers by reducing another human being to rubble. Although their legitimate desire to get down to the clinic where the patients are is understandable to sensitive faculty, relatively little has been done to make this situation possible. With the exception of a few enlightened experiments, a number of which were very costly and have not always worked well, most schools have continued to limit new students' views to what can be seen at the far end of a microscope.

Generations of medical students have found it demoralizing to trot off to medical school with certain expectations, only to find themselves doing nothing but whittling down a cadaver and repeating a lot of work they did as undergraduates. Much of the learning continues to be fun, of course, and few consider the experience a total waste. It is just a letdown to arrive thinking that at last you are going to see the sick people you have pledged your lives to cure, and then find nothing but more rats, test tubes, and the same old patient who can't talk back.

Most medical students are mature and motivated. They are smart and independent, and have excellent images of themselves. It is disillusioning for them to discover that they are confined to stools and sinks and Bunsen burners, and treated like little children. Suddenly these eager people burning for power and action and accomplishment find themselves tied down in essentially very passive learning situations with teachers who are often teachers in name only.

It is not fair to "do a number" on pre-clinical faculty across the United States, for generalizations of this kind are cruel and inaccurate. But medical educators hear so many complaints from first- and second-year students, we are obligated to have a look at the issue. Perhaps if we can understand it, *you* can deal with it a little better when your time comes to handle it.

Most teachers of the pre-clinical sciences are Ph.D. career scientists, with major interests in research in their individual fields (often narrow in focus). People being what they are, they tend to overemphasize what is of particular interest to them, and those areas in which they possess unique expertise. Just as naturally, they want their students to learn these areas well, although in the long run, these specialized interests may not be all that necessary to the making of a good general physician. A helpless captive in a powerless position, the poor freshman can do little but memorize the professor's pet project, knowing full well that it can safely be forgotten the minute the grade is in. Meanwhile, all the other tempting goodies to be learned must be sacrificed. It is enough to fire the revolutionary spirit in the meekest.

Students complain not only of the narrow interests of their professors, but also of their relative inaccessibility. They complain that they are taught, as in college, by lab assistants rather than "the big cheese." They feel rightly that they are considered unimportant by scientists high in the administrative hierarchy, who prefer to teach those who share their special interests (and who are willing to prove it by donating their time and work during elective time)!

Implicit in this feeling of being unworthy to warrant the professor's time is the realization that they are quite helpless to do anything about it without jeopardizing their positions. They can express a certain passive resistance by making jokes, neglecting their work, cheating on the material handed in, and writing condemnatory articles for the student publications. But many feelings of resentment are driven underground because there's no place for them to go.

The initial, inevitable disillusionment has become common enough that many college students are aware of what's in store before they ever set foot in medical school. The former editor of *Modern Medicine*, the late Dr. Michael Halberstam, once wrote an editorial about his response to a group of brand-new medical freshmen assigned to him for orientation. They expressed such negative attitudes, he almost didn't know how to handle the situation. In the past, he said, his job had been to deal with untempered idealism and extravagant expectation. Now he felt almost as if he had to pep up his students to convince them that medical school was really a marvelous experience and they had not made a mistake in signing up for the four year stretch.

I think it's a *good* thing that students are demanding and critical of their teachers, and urge you to be, too, when your time comes. Students who are sloughed off because they are beginners and do not ask interesting and exotic questions are actually receiving a horrendous lesson for the future. They are learning that the ordinary and uninteresting patient may be sloughed off just as they have been. Of course, it works the other way, too. People unwilling to give due recognition to the uninteresting and boring details of the basic sciences are telling patients that their interest in them is superficial and limited only to certain areas. And in medicine it is important to be able to look at problems from every standpoint.

A unique perspective on the relative merits of pure science versus the early exposure to patients has recently appeared in the medical literature. Five years ago, a man named Ludwig Eichna enrolled in medical school at the State University of New York (Downstate) in Brooklyn. Completing the four-year program successfully, he then wrote a number of articles giving his impressions of his education. He felt that the emphasis on the sciences had actually *deteriorated* and needed to be strengthened. He felt that too much attention was being given to "social" problems in medicine, which was detracting from the students' ability to concentrate on learning the substance of their profession. He criticized the loss of good lecturers, and described apprenticeship training as "bad." Flying in the face of student criticisms, he said, "During the first year, inexperienced students, eager to get at patients for self-gratification (for motivation, they say), are foisted —yes, foisted—on patients. The patients are usually not even asked whether they will allow this intrusion. . . . Titillation is not a valid reason to impose students on patients. It is also questionable whether these students learn anything of value." It is hard not to listen to these opinions with respect, for Ludwig Eichna is no ordinary doctor. He is the former chairman of the department of medicine at the very medical school from which he graduated *for the second time* in 1979. (He first graduated from the University of Pennsylvania Medical School in 1931.) What do you think of a professor who spends his retirement years going through medical school again to see it through the eyes of his students? *I* am very impressed!

Perhaps the curriculum of the first two years is indeed more dull than it needs to be, and the quality of the teaching less than desired. Nevertheless, the first two years are a time of great discovery and adventure. Every school has its superior teachers, its sympathetic lab assistants, its young Ph.D. candidates who will spend hours with students—answering their questions, helping them set up experiments, offering advice on which articles to read, shooting the breeze over 10:00 P.M. coffees.

Adventures in the lab can be the stuff of which great memories are made. During the first several years of medical school, I was able to send detailed letters of my experience home to the family and to one or two close friends. I kept copies of them, and now have only to dip into them to bring back a lot of old feelings and remembrances. Perhaps you will be able to do the same. (One of my former residents is writing a book based on journals kept in medical school, and it should be a blockbuster!) Here is living,

unedited proof that the pre-clinical years are not devoid of inspi-
rational, dedicated, pre-clinical teachers.

February 15

. . . I'm too edgy to study so I'll tell you about that
wonderful physiology department. They're just the
nicest teachers in the world. They knocked themselves out to keep things lively for us . . . including a tiny welcome sign hanging in the lab. Dr.
Hafkesbring is the head of the department, and
then there are several others, including Dr. Pincus,
who has given us most of our lectures so far. He's
an M.D., a gastro-enterologist, and a visiting lecturer in the department. He's really a doll . . .

Anyway, they have kept us stepping so, it's
unbelievable what we've done in two days. Yesterday a friend of Pincus', the head of the physiology
department at Jefferson, spent the whole day with
us. He lectured superbly, then spent hours with us
in the lab, showing us how to work with the dogs,
teaching us, answering questions, chatting infor-
mally, drawing on the blackboard. He was just
superb, and I was fascinated. He asked my lab
partner, Seana, why she wanted to be a doctor,
and told us about his 180 boys at Jefferson, and all
about his research. He's one of the top men in the
country.

Today we met Dr. somebody-or-other from Penn,
also a hoo-ha big shot with a monkey named
François with a gastric fistula and a horrible
temper. Couple of the girls got bit by rats. Mine
was the only one that died, but it wasn't my fault,
really. We gave the rats probanthine, enterogas-
trone, and histamine, and observed changes in
gastric secretion as a result of them. Then we
observed some dogs with Pavlov and Heidenhain

pouches, and the glob that came out of them. In this course you don't even get a lunch hour, just take turns taking ten minutes for a sandwich. But the spirit is marvelous!

They're friendly, they encourage millions and millions of questions, they stimulate you to think, they call themselves by their first names in front of the students, even. And Dr. Hafkesbring told me that all the physiologists in the five medical schools in the city are the same way, they all go 'round the medical schools sharing knowledge and pitching in. Boy, it's really something to see a big wheel take his tie off and roll up his sleeves and put on an apron. We studied all about saliva, gastrin, and all the other hormones and juices, etc. And we saw a fascinating movie showing a man who had half his face cut out because of a cancer and a plastic cheek put in so you could see him chew, swallow, phonate, smoke, etc. It was the most awe-inspiring demonstration I ever saw. Did you know that there are more than twenty muscles used in speaking and eating?

It is during these first two years that students come to depend upon each other for a great many things. First, they serve as guinea pigs and test objects for each other. By tradition, medical students are the most experimented upon human beings, simply because they are the most available. Who else would be willing to swallow all that stuff just to see what comes out? They go on nutrient-deficient diets to test their own metabolic reactions. They swallow drugs and record their effects. They hook themselves up to calibrating machines and watch their own heart and brain waves go rippling across a monitor.

Medical students learn how to "stick" each other, perfecting their venipuncture technique and invading each other's muscles with mutual abandon. The clumsiest usually suffer more than their victims, but everyone recognizes that this is the only way to learn, and, unfortunately, practice makes perfect. When, toward the end of their second year, they learn how to do physical examinations, their first live "patient" is their lab partner, the same one whose veins are full of holes and whose muscles are still black and blue. Medical students hot in pursuit of an intellectual challenge think nothing of demanding their classmates' bodies, specimens, and cooperative spirit. Usually they get it with good humor.

Consider the following:

> I am crazy about the wonderful people in our physiology department. We have never a dull moment . . . and some of them are not too pleasant. Today, for example, we swallowed Rehfuss tubes and I disgraced myself completely by not being able to keep the damn thing down long enough to swallow fifty cc's of 7 percent alcohol. I started out with one that had a balloon on the end for measuring duodenal motility, but the cursed animal sprang a leak and kept blowing up in my gullet while I shook with spasms of retching. Do they honestly inflict those things on *sick* people? One poor child threw up all over Dr. Pincus and his new suit; and we all laughed so hard, we nearly ended up doing the same thing ourselves. . . .

Students are continually testing their developing attitudes and opinions about their studies on their classmates and upperclassmen, using them as sounding boards and testing grounds for their reactions to life around them. Students really do learn from one another, and learning activity during those first two years is anything but isolated or antisocial. Often it is hard for students caught up in their own emotions to recognize that all others are equally affected, however diverse their overt reactions may be. Consider the following:

... Last Thursday was a more "absorbing" but less happy experience. . . . I cut up my first living animal, a dog. We worked in groups of six on intestinal absorption, and fortunately my lot fell to be "chief cook and bottle-washer" for the experiment, so I did more watching than working. I was tired and stunned in many ways when I got home. I don't know. I certainly don't seem to have the temperament of the average medical student, and I'm glad I don't. I just didn't get the pleasure out of destroying that animal that some of my fellow students seemed to feel. I was fascinated, of course, and vitally interested, but to me it was merely a means to an end; knowledge, rather than an enjoyable pastime. Not that I'm squeamish or "chicken," but I guess I'm just sensitive to some things that my cold-blooded fellow students aren't. My roommate, the "surgeon" and a terrific gal, kept the heart in formalin and blew up the lungs for a permanent mount. To me, all I could think of was that she was like a bullfighter, keeping the ears and tail. I don't think I'll ever get used to death. I can't just drop a dog in the wastebasket without digging up four years of training in the humanities, and I don't like to be teased about it either, or made to feel as if I'm "square." There's such a terrible danger in this field that one will become hardened to things which one morally should *not* become hardened to. No one has to tell me the importance of using experimental animals, I know all that; it has nothing whatsoever to do with the way I feel. I know the dog didn't "feel" anything, but *I* did! Oh, well ...

Students often tend to try to lose themselves in the crowd, taking on the protective covering of the group. Although not wishing to call attention to themselves in their insecurity, they are not shy about seeking help wherever it may be available. A student's first student is usually another student. Here's a good example of that:

> . . . In chemistry, I trudge along as I always did, keeping my mouth shut, looking unobstrusive, doing what everyone else does, and praying vigorously. I'm blessed with a roommate who knows it cold and has the faculty of imparting her knowledge to me, so that for the first time in my life, I'm learning some chemistry for *real*. If I could have had someone like her to teach me in college, chemistry need not have been the nightmare it always was for me. . . .

A medical student who has been "turned on" by a particular subject will stop at nothing to find out more. It is not uncommon for freshmen to hit the library, hot in pursuit of knowledge that is far in excess of what will be on the exam. Alternately excited and guilty, they pursue their stolen pleasures because they can't help themselves. Usually, it's exactly what their professors expect of them.

> . . . On the bright side, we heard a terrific set of lectures on the emotional effects on the G-I tract by Dr. Frank Brooks, chairman of the physiology department at the University of Pennsylvania. I was really fascinated, and ran to *Scientific American* to read the article about the "executive monkey" experiment. We also saw a movie about Wolf and Wolff's "Tom" (a man with a hole in his stomach through which his gastric processes could be observed), which was so interesting.
>
> Next Tuesday we get a speaker from England.

He is coming to Penn, and all five medical schools are invited. The last speaker who came did not know that there was a ladies' medical school in Philadelphia, and got very upset when he saw so many knowledgeable-looking females in the audience. The hapless fellow was sitting right behind Dr. Hafkesbring, our physio professor, when he said, "What in God's name are those women doing here?" Rising on her haunches, she spit fire and gall at him, saying, *"Those girls, sir, are mine!"* What a magnificent woman! And now I "gotta run." Protein and lipid test on Monday. Fooey.

One chronic state of existence to which the new medical student will need to adapt is one that he or she has already dipped into in college. It is the overwhelming feeling that there is just too much to learn, and not enough time to do it in. The pre-clinical student is deluged with often-confusing facts, details, processes, which must be mastered in sequence lest that which comes after be rendered totally unintelligible. Students complain that if they get lost anywhere during the lecture, the rest of it is Greek, and it usually is. Plunged into a sea of minutiae, most of which is not immediately relevant to anything, and soon recognizing that not all of it can be mastered, the student may be forgiven for feeling something bordering on despair and the now-familiar sense of helplessness. The all-consuming fear of failure is fueled by the unshakable belief that everyone is absorbing the material but *me!*

... We here are experiencing quite a few problems, which could well be clarified by a practitioner. Among them, how hard should a medical student work? How much of what we learn is "important"? How can we know what we will use? How do we differentiate between information that is to become an integral part of our being, how much should become reference? How much should be just familiar? How do we combat guilt over not studying enough, useless panic because others are better prepared? Is it more important to pass tests, or study for our own knowledge? How can you be objective over the terrific amount of work to be done, and our capacity for doing it? What do you do when you feel you're just not "getting" it, and more study doesn't seem to be the answer?

We all seem to be confused by things such as this and we get so much crazy advice, we really don't know what is best. We also need to know how important are the details, the trivia, which we know will be forgotten? And how is it that some girls know all the details *cold*, and other girls have children and don't work as hard and know only one fraction the amount, and yet we are all passing? Do the "A" kids make better doctors than the ones who don't know as much? What is the relationship between the book-larnin' of these two years and the lifetime that comes afterward? How can there be such a varied range of knowledge in our class, when all of us will be "doctors"? And so on and so forth!

The art of knowing what is important, and what can be left buried in reference texts until a specific need arises, is a function of growing experience. The student doesn't begin to relax until a solid feeling develops that it is OK not to have certain facts at one's fingertips, as long as he or she knows where to go to find them. Students are consoled when a kindly faculty person tells them, *"Fifty percent of everything we are teaching you is wrong . . . and we're not sure* which *fifty percent!"* It helps to be reminded that medical knowledge is constantly changing, and today's facts are tomorrow's errors, just as today's facts are also yesterday's undreamed-of cures.

Eventually, like generations of students before you, you will treat the indiscriminate digestion of facts with the contempt that it deserves. Instead, you'll be able to share the sentiments of the woman who proofread the seventh edition of Nelson's *Textbook of Pediatrics*. Evidently fed up to the teeth with the tedium of her work, she inserted an interesting item in the index. It says, *"Birds, for the, 1–1413,"* which, as you have guessed, constitutes the entire contents of the book!

Early in training, however, the pressures of keeping abreast (which are often self-imposed and unrealistic) can cause a medical student to regress to the grubby practices of his or her callow youth. It helps to recall the lessons of college days (for example, do you remember the "transience of exultation" and the "roller-coaster ego"?). Well, here's a classic example of both:

> . . . Pharmacology has me sick with fear; the exam's coming up. I have been typing my notes, making charts, quizzing the instructors, and yet I know in advance all will be to no avail. Some dope with no emotional problems will walk in there and come out 20 points ahead of me, and all the studying in the world won't be able to save me from more defeat and heartbreak. There's isn't anything I can do but sit back and wait for it to happen.

> Three weeks later
> . . . Well, I got the exam back, and lo! the village idiot came up with a big red ninety! The class average was seventy-seven, and many flunked outright! Yessir, I got an A, the eighth highest grade in a class of fifty-two. So help me God! What a stunning grade to start the new course off with! I haven't been able to figure out why I did so well. I was prepared, yes, but I've been prepared just as well for other exams where I came out on bottom. I was relatively calm and unspastic, but I have flubbed

other exams where I didn't think I was nervous.
I messed up many exams from sheer dumb bad
luck, so maybe this time I just got the breaks.
That's the only way I can figure it. But it sure
made me very happy and proud, and was a real
shot in the arm.

Or consider this perfect little scenario reflecting the blood lust
of competition (long past a career point when it is of any use
whatsoever):

. . . I got an A in my minor course, public health.
However, it didn't make a dent in my emotional
mood—no elation—purely because half the class got
A's indiscriminately, and that took the joy away
from a competitive creature like myself. Especially
when no one else in the class *deserved* an A. I can't
help these thoughts, I'm trying to be honest. . . .

. . . I'm mad because I can't be number one in the
class. It took just that one A in pharmacology to
make me realize what a terribly competitive person
I still am, and how bitterly I resent being at the
bottom of the class all the time. I wouldn't be surprised if this constant battering at my ego isn't
what keeps me feeling so full of chronic rage and
hatred all the time.

Medical students who have let their anxieties get out of hand
will pour tremendous energy into alternately defending and blaming themselves for insignificant errors. They will seek external
causes of blame inappropriately, or attempt to justify themselves
for inadequacies that are self-defined and often self-perpetuated.
In short, they can become very neurotic individuals if they don't
watch out!

Yesterday morning we got back the pathology exam which I was going to *smash* and show that D a thing or two. Well, it was an eighty-six. My first thought was to be delirious with joy. Then I found out that the class grades were very high and that very few got below a ninety! I became immediately depressed all day. You might have thought I'd gotten a sixty! Then I realized that my depression had come from anger.

I was angry with D because he had thrown a curve on the exam. Although it was on the kidney, he asked us to describe the course of events leading to hypertension in a man with an enlarged prostate, via pyelonephritis, of course. I'd long since forgotten the anatomical relations of the bladder. I put down that it obstructed the ureters, but of course it was the urethra, and he took off six points. After I had studied and knew such minutiae about the *kidney!* So I was mad at him.

Then I was mad at my classmates because, although I had studied harder than most of them, they had all managed to do better than I. I hated them because most of them had been sharp enough to dig up his favorite questions from the past and prepare them specifically. So, some kids who knew less than I did better by looking up the answer the night before.

Last, I was mad at myself for having failed to be as slick as the others. So I was raging at the world. When I realized what I was doing, I stopped. But what is a better way to handle it all?

One of the major tasks of a medical student is to learn "a better way to handle it all." The attempt to do so is part of the process called "taking oneself apart and putting oneself back together again" mentioned in Chapter Five. It is a task that *must* be accomplished if students are to free themselves from fear, guilt, and anxiety. Unfortunately, not everyone accomplishes this easily or without help.

The newsletter of the American Medical Student Association recently quoted John Henry Pfifferling, Ph.D., who had been studying stress in medical education, and running workshops to relieve it.

> Fear, anxiety, and frustration pervade the lives of medical students, a tight feeling in the chest dominates their existence. It is usually associated with dread that they may injure a patient in the process of learning to be healers, or that they may fail in their attempts to become physicians. . . . Students are debilitated by their own "mistake fantasies" and they are often troubled by a "disquieting rage." . . . Students uniformly expressed fear, guilt and anxiety. . . .

I believe there are at least two major impediments to speedy resolution of the problems of pre-clinical medical students, both of them superimposed upon them by "the system," and therefore less easy to remedy than those anxieties born of personal adjustments. The first of these we have already touched upon, the "infantilization" of grown persons who also happen to be students (traditionally a child's role, remember).

Students frustrated by the demands of their dead patient, and the staggering work load of all the laboratory courses whose content does not appear to be too relevant to their ultimate purpose, are right to complain that they are infantilized. The "Prussian army" model of medical school demands that the good little soldiers obey the rules, toe the line, absorb the material, make no flack, voice no dissension, and rock no boats. (After all, someday they will be leaders and healers of men!) Because the setting is a "school," which runs on classrooms, teachers, semesters, exams, and the like, people seem to forget that the kiddies and future generals have grown up, and have learned how to think for themselves. They tire of their continuing roles as desk-sitters and hand-raisers. Students hate continuing their old patterns of exam-worrying, grade-chasing, classmate-watching, brown-nosing, and nail-biting. They succumb to the discipline with poor grace, often giving the very erroneous impression that they just don't like to work as hard as they used to in "the old days."

The second force mitigating against successful resolution of the medical student quakes is the phenomenon I once referred to as "Terror on the Training Ground," in a column with that title. Now we are no longer dealing with the nature and form of the learning process, or the resurgence of "grubby practices" in response to stress, but rather with shabbily unhelpful attitudes and practices among certain faculty members. Some of them can be absolutely rotten to students who are in no position to fight back. There are times when students are treated so callously and with such indifference to their human suffering, one cannot help but ask if there isn't a covert tradition among some faculty to haze a student, or force him or her to prove worth as a physician in a totally unnecessary way.

There are sadistic people in every walk of life, fortunately very few. But they exert a negative influence far out of proportion to their numbers, particularly when they are in positions of power. It is hard when they have too stringent goals and ideals for students, for they cause them grief if they do not measure up. Some have not surmounted their own prejudices against certain students, making them pay a personal penalty for faults that are apparent to no one else. Minority students are particularly vulnerable to these individuals, as are women, but all suffer from their unresolved personal problems.

In "Terror on the Training Ground," I undertook a discussion of people of this kind, citing a number of real examples of abuse. I was surprised that it evoked so many letters from physicians who retained wretched memories of their own persecution as under-graduates. It was so bad, I immediately had to run back to the typewriter to grind out a companion piece that told only of the loving, kind, and wonderful faculty who had existed side by side with the brutes.

Here are some excerpts from letters written to me by people who felt they had experienced the nether side of medical education:

> From a faculty member in Wisconsin:
> . . . Your article this month struck me even more than usual. I guess this is because I have been teaching H---- here for twenty years (after being teaching assistant in pre-meds at C---- University for four), and grew up academically in the tradition that you so well describe. For many years, I was one of the deliverers of the hazing, and have lived through the painful process of rebirth into in-creased concern for the people who are becoming doctors. One result is that I have just been ap-pointed the assistant dean for student affairs, with primary responsibility for students in the first two years. The opportunities feel very exhilarating right now, as I have the mandate to look for ways to humanize the experiences of the students in those years. The more I have looked at the prob-lems, the more I have been struck with the dehu-manizing life experiences of much of the faculty; and I am concentrating some of my efforts in seek-ing ways to help the faculty find their own human-ity, which has so long been hidden from them. It's been a long, hard process for me, this trying to grow myself from within while faced with de-humanizing experiences and a reputation among students that seemed to take forever to change.

From a practitioner in Virginia:

... I can't begin to tell you what a resonant note [your article] struck with me ... ah, how familiar everything you described sounded to me. This psychological degradation going on, which is as real as it can be, really concerns me. I think that it degrades the quality of the education which is potentially available—at least it certainly did for me. And I don't think that it is at all necessary, or even constructive in building "character."

... I went to the University of -----, and graduated in 1969. It was the most miserable and despicable four years of my life. ... I very seldom discuss this with people, for it is very unbecoming to seem bitter, when one should feel warmth and gratitude to one's mother of learning. And I am not a griper. I have enjoyed everything else, every other institution—jobs, internship, residencies, college, prep school, friends, duties—I have always managed to find my happiness in these and think that I will for the future. But, ah, medical school. There is a bitterness I will hold in my heart for the rest of my life. I have never been under the thumb of a more Calvinistic, sadistic group of people in my life.

... The long, tiring hours and physical exhaustion that I was able to endure with a rather stoic outlook. I thought that it was an anachronism, even the forces of economics taking advantage of the bottom man on the totem pole, but I never felt bitter about it. ... But the mental cruelty, which gave many faculty members obvious delight! About that I am bitter. I never met one M.D. in medical school who seemed to be a happy person, or who enjoyed medicine. It was only after I got out into the real world that I ever finally met my first Doc who seemed to be a joyous man and a warm human being. I suspected that such people existed while in medical school, but knew that I would never find them in those ivy-covered halls. . . . I have eventually learned—with no help from my professors, thank you—that medicine can be very fulfilling and inspiring. . . . In a more constructive sense, I have often wondered, no, hoped, that it might be possible to help future medical students avoid this, to some extent. . . .

From a woman physician in Philadelphia:
. . . You asked readers who felt moved to share their experiences with you to do so. I'd like to recount just a few of my own humiliations to you. My first week of medical school, my histology professor found out that I had two children. He asked me in front of my whole lab section what the hell I thought I was doing in medical school with two children and didn't I know anything about birth control. . . . Just last week in a psychiatry class, with twenty-seven men and two women, I was asked to discuss how I would feel about having a mastectomy. And so it goes on—still thoughtless or cruel or humiliating. I hope someday we will be able to train doctors *humanely*. . . .

If you haven't spent enough time contemplating the years of study required before your state board of medicine will let you become the licensed physician you want to be, you'd do well to stop at this point and ask yourself, "Hey, do I really want to be a doctor *that* badly? Who needs it? Do I really want to be one of the 16 percent of medical students living on tranquilizers? Or one of the 15 percent on amphetamines, the 25 percent on pot, or the 10 percent on booze? Will I become one of the 30 percent in counseling, or one of the 90 percent who need it? Do I want to be one of those stressed-out freaks whose suicides are second only to accidents as their cause of premature death?"

It's no use. I might as well save my breath. I know there's not a word I can say that would make you feel any differently about a career in medicine, so I might as well go on.

There are a number of coping mechanisms that medical students have used for years, and you can learn them, too. Once the first half of your training is over, those six years in "school," you'll be well on your own. Here are some of them.

The first one is *complaint*. Complaining is a positive commandment for medical students. It is so therapeutic no one could possibly survive without periodically raising it to a high art form. Dr. Ned Cassem, in a very compassionate and funny address ("Internship, Liberty, Death, and Other Choices: How to Survive Life in a Hospital") to graduating seniors at Harvard Medical School several years ago, gave guidelines and suggestions on ostentatious and articulate complaining. In support of his philosophy, "Run away sometimes, hate often, complain constantly," he suggests. "When the [warning] signal lights on your own psychic instrument panel light up, you are being hit. . . . When you are hit, holler. . . . To insure this you need your peer group. Stick together. Loners get hit harder. Women take heed, you are at higher risk. You have full complaining rights with the same full vocabulary. The group should be a good in-house Paranoid Club; let no one hear you except those who understand. Remember you are not in a club to change anything, you are there to complain. Do it creatively. Imaginary retaliation is better than none. Finally, when you've been especially creative (for instance, you've come up with a Turkey Scale for Private Attendings), keep it anonymous. . . ." What an uproarious and helpful speech that was!

Now I'll share one of *my* last letters with you, If Nobel prizes were awarded for griping, this one should surely qualify. Take note—the last line provides the clue to the letter's *real* agenda.

This is going to be another futile, hopeless, un-answerable letter, and I have no valid reason for writing it, but I'm doing it anyway.

I have a bacteriology final on Saturday morning. I had the whole day off to study but accomplished nothing. I am very resistant. I don't want to study. I am sick of medical school. I wish I had never heard of it with all my heart and soul. I am so bored and sick and fed up to the teeth with stupid, uninteresting, unnecessary, unrememberable minu-tiae, I could take the whole course and stick it right up the professors' respective asses one by one.

I don't see any point to the whole business. I don't know what I am doing here; I obviously will never know enough to practice medicine and I wish to even less. I would much rather be out at the movies, or the theater, or a concert, or an art gallery, or a zoo, or with a good book, or out for a ride in the country, or visiting congenial friends, or even going to a good lecture, or working on some useful, interesting, productive work that has noth-ing to do with medicine.

I don't give a shit if I flunk straight out. I will probably get a D in bacteriology because I studied only six pages *all day* and I don't care one hoot. I am sick and tired of stuffing useless shit down my throat. Life is one long, terrible, horrible grind, and I don't care if I get kicked out. *I just do not care*!!!! That is final. I'm not going to whine any more about studying and not getting anywhere. I frankly am *not going to study* and anything that happens is my own fault.

Well, maybe I *do* still have to go back to work, but nobody can make me like that crap and I am only going to learn the *bare minimum* because I *hate* it. I'm *sick sick sick sick sick of medical school.* I'm sick of anxiety and worry and not being prepared, and taking notes and studying notes, and flaming loops and switching to high power, and cutting up corpses and trying not to vomit in surgery rounds, and not having enough time to take tea in the morning and watching rabbits convulse, and writing a lot of *crap* down in a lot of notebooks and laughing at D's feeble jokes and taking *goddam* examinations!

I'm sick of going to school at 8:30 every morning and coming home at 5:00 at night and studying all evening. I'm sick of not going out and having fun and meeting people and talking to people and dating people. I'm sick of hanging on the mailbox to see who loves me today and counting days to a weekend when I will have the pleasure of calling home as my treat for the week. I'm sick of trying to understand myself and fighting anxiety and depression and misery and not getting anywhere. I'm *sick sick sick* of my stupid, philistine, insensitive roommates whom I cordially despise.

I'm sick of being alive. I'm sick of being in the same horrible, terrible rut with no future and no past, and nothing to look forward to with hope and nothing to look back on but regret that I haven't handled things better. I'm sick of living each grim, sordid, stupid, unending day at a time when it's been hundreds of days since anything *happy* and *sweet* and *really good* has happened to me. I'm sick of feeling trapped, frightened, inadequate, and alone. I'm sick of trying to make the goddam contact lenses stay in for more than an hour. I'm sick and tired of trying to keep happy when I'm *not*, goddam it, and don't have any reason to be. I'm sick of futilely trying to keep from gaining weight. I'm sick of my appearance which reflects how I feel; I'm sick of my hair which won't grow. I'm sick of thinking, "I'm never going to be a practicing doctor because I'll never be any good." I'm sick of my foggy brain and headaches, and lack of memory, and dullness and stupidity and being at the bottom of a class of morons. I'm sick of the rat race. Anything else? Oh, yes, *and I'm sick of you!* Now I have to get back and study.

The second approach is a *sense of humor.* Medical students are famous for their ability to lasso the ludicrous. Most of this is gallows humor, but some of it is just plain Abbott and Costello. Here's one example.

> . . . Feeling was pretty strong about the bacteriology exam yesterday. Everyone had studied furiously and it was the kind of test where it just didn't help. Anyway, everyone in the class showed up in black today as a gag, no make-up, no jewelry, as a protest of mourning for our lost grades. It was enormously effective. We looked like fifty black crows in the lecture room. The deans and professors split their sides laughing at us. It was a good release for me (but the brooding trouble is still there and so is my terrible headache . . .).

A brooding sense of trouble or a headache *can* be expelled, nevertheless, by a proper attitude and a chance to let off steam. (OK, this time it didn't work!) At my school we had an annual event called Skit Night, at which the four classes put on twenty-minute musical playlets that savaged the faculty and made up for our months of pressure. No holds were barred, and professorial victims had to take it with good grace. We lived off the afterglow for weeks. Make it your business to do the same.

Another coping mechanism is the attempt to *deal directly* with the misery. More and more medical schools are developing "human potential" groups for students. They are an outgrowth of the movement that originated on the rocky coast of California, and often work well. Physicians are desperately in need of the opportunity to talk to themselves about what they are going through. Dr. Michael Balint, a British psychiatrist, offered some of his colleagues the opportunity to do just that, and similar groups here have sprung up to deal with these needs. Most deal with the physicians' attitudes and feelings toward patients. However, even undergraduates could use a place where they could say what they feel, knowing that the understanding of peers makes the process safe for honest disclosure. We never had anything like that, and, believe me, we all could have used it.

Finally, medical students need *hope*. The best expression of that is to buy yourself a good stethescope months before you'll need it; order some of those short white jackets in anticipation of the time when you can give up your long white lab coat; and get yourself a little M.D. medallion for the rear bumper of your car. The cops won't honor it for parking violations, but, boy, it sure looks good tucked in the glove compartment. No one has to know that you bought it!

8.
Patients, at Last (The Clinical Years)

It has not been easy so far to give you anything but an impressionistic picture of the first six years, because, as you can appreciate, there are many variables. No two schools are alike, nor are any two students. Some student doctors breeze through the experience, utterly unflappable and always ready to have some fun, and others seem particularly sensitive to the issues I have been raising for your consideration.

Do you think you are in a better position to evaluate the future at this point? Do you have any ideas about how you would tackle the challenges that have been presented? Do you know what kind of a student *you* will be when your time comes? If not, make no premature judgments. Read on.

I promised you back in Chapter Three that if you'd read the material on the pre-clinical years with a grain of salt, a sense of humor, and an open mind, it would all get better. And the time has really come. A new sense of electricity and excitement comes into a sophomore class in medical school as the spring approaches. It will not be long before work begins on the wards, and patients are no longer unattainable objects, but flesh-and-blood partners in the learning process.

No longer will patients be recognized only by their specimens. The time is over for students to study microscope slides of livers and spleens; gallon jugs of urine stored in the fridge like apple cider; incubated plates of sputum streaked onto growth media; long bones pinned with wires to ball and socket joints; distended organs shipped over from the week's most exciting autopsy. No longer are patients transformed into print and flattened into pages of textbooks a thousand pages thick. Now the patient is put back together like a thoroughly reconditioned typewriter from IBM, and the student is invited to come over to the hospital to pinch and poke him while he is still breathing and possessed of all his bits and parts relatively intact.

Patients are fun, more fun than a barrel of monkeys. They are the pot of gold at the end of the student's climb up the rainbow. And no one is more eager to tackle them than the third-year upperclassman who has earned their regard by surviving.

The third-year student may be defined as that irrepressible human being who, for some incomprehensible reason, still wants to be a doctor after all he's* been through. He's been given six years to recognize the folly of his ways and transfer over to the Stanford School of Business, whose MBA would enable him to start out at more money than he could someday make as a sixth-year, postgraduate medical fellow. But the mad, obsessed fool still wants to get his itchy hands on patients, and drive home every night with a Littmann stethescope slung oh so casually around his neck.

Perhaps he has too much invested in his dream to quit now. Perhaps he has become so adept at mastering the collegiate "grubby practices" he now eats them for dinner. Perhaps he's been getting such a bang out of his studies he wants more. No

---

* At this point in my manuscript, I am succumbing to the rigidity of the English language and choosing a sex for my narrative. I just can't deal with that "him or her" and "she/he" business any more. In the interests of keeping thoughts flowing, I have decided to cop out and go with the majority. I hope the sentiments I express will be more nonsexist than my language.

longer interviewing and examining selected patients under supervision, or sitting passively in the audience while the most interesting are presented publicly, the student doctor is now assigned his
very own sick people to "work up" and submit to treatment programs. He would have been a dope to transfer over to another
profession; he's about to have the time of his life!

Most upperclassmen prepare for their first meeting with a patient by a visit to the uniform store. The medical student balls up
his long white lab coat and chucks it, replete with two years'
worth of stains and holes, into the rag bin instead of the laundry.
In its place, he slips into the short white jacket of the clinical physician. What a high!

On its left lapel, he sticks the ambiguously worded identification pin that says "Dr. John Smith." In the lower *right*-hand
pocket (this is highly ritualized), he places his twice-folded
stethescope, with just the right amount of earpiece protruding
from the top. In the lower *left*-hand pocket, he stuffs his black-
leather, mini-loose-leaf binder, with empty leaves on which he'll
record patients' vital statistics, and the tables that will give him normal laboratory values, customary dosages of common drugs, met-
ric conversion factors, a calendar-horoscope, and whatever else
this year's printers have thrown in to amuse him during tedious
clinical conferences.

His breast pocket will be crammed with a reflex hammer, a tun-
ing fork, a flashlight, some ballpoint pens, a bunch of keys, a
chewed-up package of Lifesavers, and something like a tissue on
top to keep the whole mess from falling out whenever he bends
over to pick up something that already *has*. Tucked under his
arm, or trotting along beside him, is his trusty little black bag,
containing, above all else, his *Merck Manual* (or a reasonable imitation). This handy scout guide will condense everything he has
ever learned about disease into unreadable print, and make it
readily available when he gets into a jam and has to duck into a
corner to find out what to do quick.

As he approaches the assigned room, and is about to enter it for
the first time solo, he exhibits characteristic signs of excitement,

nervousness, and anticipation. His heart is beating double time, his palms are wet, his tongue cleaves to the roof of his mouth, and his mind becomes as blank as an erased tape. In other words, he's in *fine* shape to interview and examine his first patient.

The hospital patient waiting behind closed doors may be defined as a suffering human being of variable age, sex, character, personality, and symptoms. He, or statistically more likely *she*, is wearing night clothes in broad daylight. She is stretched out or doubled up on a bed or stretcher in some acute form of bodily or mental distress. If conscious, she is possessed of a facial expression that clearly asks the student, "Who are you? What are you doing here? Better still, what am *I* doing here? Are you going to hurt me?" (If the student is paranoid, he'll imagine that she is also thinking, "Why is your tongue sticking to the roof of your mouth, dummy?")

In this encounter is all of medicine. Of course, there are infinite variations to the two players described here, and the situations in which they find themselves. The patient may be asymptomatic and puzzled, too sick to talk, too distraught to give a coherent history, too hostile to cooperate with anyone, too young or too old to respond. The student may be more or less gifted at interviewing, examining, and dealing with problem situations. But what follows is medicine in a nutshell.

Since one of the purposes of this book is to get a handle on the critical issues you'll be dealing with in school, let's turn now to the challenges arising in the *clinical*, or "patient," years. There are many, and they are different from those of the first six years. Virtually all relate to the fact that, from now on, you will be dealing not only with *yourself*, the object, the student, but with *him*, the subject, the patient. Therefore, your major challenge will no longer be your own survival and endurance, but *his*. Your success or failure will hinge no longer on how *you* feel, but on how *he* feels. The transition is not automatic, for your capacity to understand and serve another human being may not be related directly to your capacity to understand, serve, or beat down on yourself.

Put it this way. The major task of a *pre-clinical* student is to build a fund of scientific knowledge, acquire technical expertise, and gain a theoretical and comprehensive awareness of the normal and abnormal processes that afflict human beings. In the mastery of this material, he must often master himself as well. The major task of the *clinical* student is to relate this encyclopedic knowledge to the needs of one single individual. This channeling down from the global and encyclopedic to the concrete and highly specific cannot be accomplished without the capacity to relate to the patient as intently as the student used to relate to himself. Patients cannot be mastered by sheer force of will; they must be *understood*. The best students are those who can understand as well as master themselves, for the patient reaps the benefit of both.

Sir William Osler is properly revered by the medical profession for having introduced bedside teaching as the heart of the medical educational experience. He knew that students can learn only a limited amount from textbooks and must treat live human beings to make their academic knowledge crystallize. But it is not easy! The medical student who formerly related exclusively to the library, laboratory, teacher, and classroom (where he could establish his own limitations on intimacy) must now confront a wretched stranger alone in a room—and find out what the hell is going on with him. This transition, difficult under the best of circumstances, is unspeakable when the patient has had a stroke and cannot talk, knows no English, is too sick to communicate, or comes from a racial, ethnic, age, or sex group that triggers negative emotions in the student.

The student doctor quickly learns that the lessons in his sophomore physical diagnosis course gave only a mechanic's knowledge of how to take a history or do a physical. Since the patient is not an engine, the stethoscope is not a pair of pliers, and the student is not yet Dr. Goodwrench, what is he supposed to do *now*? Historically, the academic assumption has been that the well-trained student will quickly take hold and gain experience to supplement those rudimentary lectures of the previous spring. Time and continued study will teach him which questions to ask, which leads to follow, which signs or symptoms indicate the need to obtain immediate substantiation of his diagnostic hunches. And that's exactly what happens.

Unfortunately, it is not enough. There's more to patient interaction than what can be learned in the medical toolshed, automotive garage, or test kitchen. Students certainly need to emphasize the acquisition of facts, objective criteria of disease, demonstrable signs of illness, and "hard" symptoms. But they also need to learn how to hear what patients are saying, how to listen between the lines. They need to know how to facilitate confidences by patients, and how to provide a climate that will enhance the interchange between them. They must learn to understand the subjective feelings that are operating as the "objective" facts are garnered, feelings that influence and distort all those classic textbook descriptions of disease. Yet in most schools, students are rarely taught how to determine the "hidden agenda" of each interview, or how to establish the emotional bonds that will decide the ultimate success or failure of the encounter.

As you read this, you may wonder how well *you* would do at talking to patients and eliciting their innermost fears and secrets. Perhaps your conviction that you would be good at this is one of the reasons you've been considering medicine. And certainly you have classmates who wouldn't consider a career as a doctor simply because they know they *couldn't* handle it. The fact remains that even native empathy can be enhanced by the acquisition of interpersonal skills and techniques, which *can* be taught. I think that more and more schools are starting to offer this material in formal courses. (Certainly the residency programs in family practice are allocating funds and teaching time to it.) They recognize the importance of helping the student doctor view the patient with the proper "detached concern."

Perhaps you've heard that each time medical students study a new disease, they think they have it. There really exists an interesting and funny phenomenon in which occasionally a student reads a description of Wotchmacallit's disease and says to himself,

"Hmm! Tiredness, pallor, nausea, fine rash over the hands, itching of the earlobes in cold weather. . . . Why, that's just what I've been complaining of for the past few weeks!" He goes over to inspect his complexion in the bathroom mirror, examines his palms under the desk lamp, and promptly goes into a panic—particularly if Wotchmacallit's disease is always fatal. When sanity returns, he's able to reassure himself that his earlobes have been itching in cold weather for twenty years, the nausea was probably the lobster, and since he isn't dead by now, he probably doesn't have W's disease after all. Needless to say, he's ashamed of his foolishness and relieved that he didn't share his suspicions with any of his classmates, or they'd tease him unmercifully. Then he picks up Harrison's *Textbook of Medicine* and moves on to Hoozeewotzi's syndrome (which he may develop, too). He's exhibited a classic case of identification with the patient; a bit overdone, of course, but proof positive that he's on his way to becoming a doctor who can translate textbook data into sensible reality judgments.

It is necessary and proper for a medical student to be able to *empathize with* a patient; that is, to be able to imagine himself in the patient's place and understand what he is thinking and feeling. It may also be useful for him to be able to *identify with* the patient, and feel that they share one or more common bonds. One of the first tasks of the clinical student, however, is to keep from *overidentifying with* the patient, for that can cause him emotional anguish and color his judgment, neither of which is in the best interest of either party.

I'm sure you have already deduced that the inability to keep a certain distance is a potential danger, and, indeed, it is what turns some people completely off the idea of even becoming a doctor. ("Oh, I could never be a doctor; I'd be all upset over anybody who was dying!") It is a skill that can be learned, but it is a great challenge, and people do not always succeed. If the job is not accomplished well, it will leave the young physician appearing calloused and hardened toward his patients. Sometimes, he is such a softie, he simply has to cover up his true feelings by being abrupt, curt, and inappropriately matter-of-fact. We have all known physicians who dealt with their fear, sorrow, and horror in this way, and we don't like them very much, perhaps unfairly.

Medical students who are able to talk about their feelings when first confronted with severely upsetting patients tell us frankly that they felt like bursting into tears, or running out of the room, or even throwing up all over the patient. Some of them have even done so. For many, dealing with their actions afterward is almost as difficult as the initial "lapse." It is important for us to reassure them that their reactions are natural in beginners, that they betray a kind heart rather than a childish one, and that they can grow to understand and moderate their feelings and the way they react to patients.

You may never know how you will feel or behave until you are confronted with an actual situation, although you are probably speculating even now about how you would "measure up." (There you go, behaving like a self-judgmental medical student already!)

You must also remember that not everyone reacts to every kind of patient the same way. Consider the pediatric oncologists, who spend their entire professional lives treating children with cancer. They have the capacity to walk peacefully into a waiting room full of heartbreaking little children whose hair has fallen out due to their chemotherapy. Other physicians become anesthesiologists, whose patient contact is limited to a pre-op visit to make sure the patient isn't allergic to a proposed induction agent, and a post-op check to make sure he's fully awake and responsive. A rare few students early in their careers feel challenged by the diseases of old age and a special warmth for the helpless elderly. Others flee these "unrewarding" patients and restrict their practices to young athletes who require nothing more than the repair of a torn cartilege or a scratching of their jogger's itch. Pathologists can go for thirty years without physically laying eyes on patients, although they work with their diseased organs every day. Obstetricians, who are supposedly the "happy" doctors, have a bad time when an obstetrical patient dies—it is usually a young woman at what is a high point in her life, until the fatal moment when everything goes wrong. Public-health physicians are traditionally grandiose types who want to fix the world, and they become impatient chained to an office grinding out patients by the hour while larger issues remain unsolved. It is safe to say that increasing experience, and an openness to one's own developing needs and interests, will help a student resolve which way he wants to go. The beginning of specialty choices based on the kinds of patients one most enjoys working with begins fairly early.

Even if one has been emotionally overwhelmed by a patient, a student doctor is not defenseless. There are ways to learn how to deal with patients in which the patient is not harmed, and the doctor is protected. We'll talk more about it later, but here's one small example. I received some very stunning advice once from one of my anatomy professors, the same gentleman who flipped his cork because we had destroyed the *palmaris longus.* Calling me aside one day, he said, "Miss Bluestone, you really have got to learn how to control your face!" "I beg your pardon?" I asked, very puzzled. "Well," he explained, "everything you think shows on your face—your confusion, your disagreement, your bewilderment. You can't let everything show like that. Someday you'll be talking to patients, and you may not want them to know what you are thinking. You have to learn to control your face!" It was a bit inappropriate for a woman who was up to her eyeballs in the musculo-skeletal system, but I never forgot his admonition. I made a conscious effort over the next few years to practice maintaining an impassive exterior, and to the extent that I succeeded (not very well), it clearly worked to everyone's advantage. Poker players would make good doctors, for they have the option of sharing only what they wish, and not what their instincts betray.

In dealing with patients, incoming juniors find that they must deal with problems other than simply the disease processes that are doing their numbers on the patient's belly or chest or brain. We're speaking now about pain, disability, disfigurement, and other by-products of the disease itself.

Pain is a frightening phenomenon to witness, particularly when it is not easily controlled, or occurs in an especially vulnerable patient with whom we closely identify. I remember sewing up policemen and firemen in the emergency room without too much trouble, for they were tough and brave, full of jokes and defiant in the face of pain. (This didn't stop some of them from keeling over from a needle stick!) A fragile little old lady with the pain of cancer, however, would almost bring tears to my eyes.

Fortunately, most pain can be alleviated, and doing so is one of the new physician's most rewarding activities. When the relief is dramatic and swift, the good feelings are, too. One example of this? Well, adult males may suddenly develop an inability to urinate after surgery or because of some lower urinary tract obstruction. The simple act of passing a catheter up the passageway can relieve a distended bladder and turn a man with agonizing pain into a smiling little kid who's ready to turn over and drift off into a healing sleep.

Sometimes it is necessary to *cause* pain, to temporarily hurt a patient for a greater good. Perhaps the patient has no veins accessible to receive an IV and must undergo a small "operation" to get one open. Causing pain to relieve pain, or to prolong or save life, is but one of the many paradoxes of medicine with which a junior student must begin to come to grips.

Disability is another painful phenomenon with which to deal, particularly when it occurs in someone who is uniquely handicapped by the disability. It is shocking to confront a young quadriplegic for the first time! So often it is a handsome teenager who tried one twist too many from a poorly sprung diving board; or a young soldier who got hit before he knew what hit him, and will remember his particular war longer than any of his buddies. Hemi- or quadriplegia even happens to pianists, artists, and others who are entitled to feel devastated when it strikes! Surprisingly, the best therapists are often the patients themselves, who teach other patients and professional staff alike what courage is, and who set incredibly moving examples for people who define life by use of limbs.

Disfigurement is an aesthetic tragedy that can shock a new physician as badly as a severe disability. When a young girl's face is cut by a razor, knife, or flying glass, everyone feels a particular pang, and works with fingers inspired to do their most exquisite repair work. Severe burns are particularly rough to handle at first. I remember dreading fresh cases, for they were so devastating in appearance and prognosis; other doctors felt especially challenged by them, because so much knowledge and skill was required to save lives, appearances, and functions. Surgical and radiation disfigurement, which is physician-induced (iatrogenic), is very much a topic for public discussion today. The prime example of this is breast surgery. Accusations that physicians are insensitive to the effects of mutilating surgery, or may even take a perverse pleasure in removing women's breasts, strike me as being tremendously unfair to physicians who, if anything, are *obsessed* with doing a good job. Undoubtedly, you have your own opinions on the subject.

It can't be stressed often enough that dealing with one's feelings about certain kinds of patients and problems is something that grows on the job. A student who comes onto the surgical service for the first time is given the task of changing simple dressings. Often they are dripping and stinking with pus, and running to nauseating colors. He wouldn't be human if he didn't keep his lips tightly closed to keep his retching under control. With his nostrils shut off and his lips sealed, he'll probably be breathing through his ears for the first few days, but in no time he will become an old pro, and honestly *mean* it when he removes a pile of old gauze and says of the healing wound, "Hey, man, that's looking absolutely gorgeous this morning!"

Disease, disability, and disfigurement all offer some hope for positive intervention. In some cases the physician may cure, in some cases he may offer relief or improvement. In all cases, we hope he would offer comfort. (One often-quoted old medical maxim states that at the least, he should do no harm!) One important task for the student now is to learn what he realistically can offer, how to scale his expectations appropriately, to be grateful for what he can do, and to avoid punishing himself for what he cannot. (That includes useless rumination about how well someone else may have functioned given the circumstances.) These are not easy things to learn. Students meet patients they care deeply about, and who trigger the most intolerable feelings of impotence, helplessness, grief, and doubt. Among these we number most often the dying.

Volumes, encyclopedias have been written about death and dying, from the perspective of the patient, the family, and the health-care professional, as well as from medical ethicists who view it from on high.

Confronting *death* is probably the single most painful and difficult task a student has to face, especially when the patient is young, attractive, and dying a particularly senseless or useless death. (As if *any* death had "meaning.") American students raised to a sense of entitlement about a long life sometimes suffer more than those from cultures who have witnessed death often, and are supported by religious and philosophical beliefs that soften the blow.

(In fact, this can also cause them problems, here. One of my classmates as an intern was a Chinese woman who had been educated in the Philippine Islands. Called to see a dying elderly patient during the night, she did not come until morning, by which time the patient had already expired. Summarily dismissed and given just twenty-four hours to remove her silks from her closet, she was utterly baffled at the uproar. "The patient was old and going to die anyway," she said before she left.)

Students handle their feelings in many ways. Some see dying patients as temples of the enemy. They hate that enemy Death so much, they appear willing to destroy its temple along with it. Without supervision, patients get blitzed and leveled like classical monuments destroyed by conquerors to make building blocks for the new architecture. Others deny the impending event in less spectacular ways. Some are able to go about the work of treatment to prolong life, palliate, provide comfort and relief from suffering as a means of making themselves feel better about what they cannot control. Some overidentify and suffer; of these, many will neglect their dying patients because contact is so painful.

You will handle this as well as any, when your time comes.

In addition to dealing with pain, disability, disfigurement, dying, and death itself, there are other major emotional challenges to the student physician.

One of them is *dealing with patients who present behavioral problems* above, beyond, or directly connected to their physical ailments. A junior student need be on the wards no longer than a week before he loses some of the romantic notions he has nourished all those years about the delightful character of sick people. He discovers that patients cannot be counted upon to be grateful, obliging, cooperative, intelligent, compliant, worshiping, or even minimally admiring. Illness and discomfort may have made them whining, complaining, tyrannical, ungrateful, critical, obstructive, hostile, or even direct agents of sabotage. Perhaps they were *always* unlikable people! Every ward has its chronic repeaters because of noncompliance, unrepentant hypochondriacs, noncooperative troublemakers, and borderline crazies, who drive the nurses to drink, try the endurance of their roommates, and make the doctors want to discharge them through the nearest window. Every pediatrics unit has its "spoiled brats" and screamers, its tantrum-throwers and ink-spillers. Every geriatrics ward has its old men who toilet on the floor whenever it has been freshly washed, and its little old ladies who become fecally incontinent the very day their discharge orders have been written, and there's no way it was just an accident.

A doctor is in trouble if he cannot learn to handle the patient who makes him want to scream. The doctor has so much power at his disposal, so many ugly threats he can legitimately make, so many unpleasant sanctions he can dutifully impose, he is honor-bound to be able to abort harsh and punitive behavior that could masquerade as treatment were he less honest. Some people, even as young medical students, have the patience of saints (although this is more characteristically an attribute of nurses). Others have to find constructive outlets for their anger, and ways of coming to terms with "the miserable patient."

Another area of potential problems lies not with the patient, but with *the patient's family*. An intelligent, cooperative, supporting family can ease the student's load tremendously. But what are one's duties and responsibilities when the patient is a dear, lovely woman saddled with a family that is loathsome? Examples are legion. Husbands of perfectly strong, capable wives beg the student not to tell them that they have cancer, fearing an hysterical outburst that is actually just a specter, and is really an insult to the woman in question. Wives, on the other hand, will persecute the nurses because they have not been quick enough to respond to their husband's call bell, usually for a minor request initiated by the wife. Geriatricians spend countless hours fending off overprotective, interfering children, who are usually compensating with secondary guilt for years of perceived or unrecognized neglect. Pediatricians good-naturedly complain that the only hard part of their profession is dealing with the mommies.

Not all families are problems, of course, and when they are, they are also part of the solution. But even under the best of circumstances, learning to deal with them, and the appropriate involvement of them in the patient's care, is a major task. Many never learn to accomplish this adequately, for the issues involved are a complicated mix of psychology, ethics, and circumstance.

Think for a minute about your own memories of the times *you* went to the doctor, and were helped or hindered by the presence of your mother, or some other adult figure. These memories will be brushing the corners of your mind as you start to deal with your own patients. Volumes have been written about the "doctor-patient relationship," that sanctified connection that has been the core of medicine since the days of the legendary Hippocrates on the Greek isle of Cos (back in the golden age of Greece). A doctor's first responsibility is to his patient, and it is to this person alone that he owes allegiance, the confidentiality of his disclosures, the privacy of his findings, and sole responsibility in decision making. But people do not live in a vacuum any more now than they did in classical times. How *should* a physician interact with a spouse, parent, or child so that the patient will get well or be controlled as quickly and easily as possible? How much should he tell? How should it be done? And when? When the doctor enlists the family's aid, is he betraying a trust? And what happens when, as often happens, both occur at the same time? If a man comes to the doctor with a venereal disease, should the doctor tell the wife so that she can protect herself and be treated—and thus betray his patient's confidence?

Families have been known to come between a patient and his doctor in the most unconscionable way, planting seeds of doubt about the latter's capabilities in the mind of a sick person who is in no position to be dealing with it at such a time. (Sometimes they are right, which complicates the issue even further.) On the other hand, they have been known to intervene successfully to make a patient more cooperative, thus ensuring the success of treatment. How should these families be addressed?

The now-familiar ogre of "not enough time" also obscures a doctor's relationship with the patient's family. How much time should legitimately be spent in building bridges and establishing communication with a family, when crowds of other patients are in need? When there are five anxious children crowding around the hallways, must the doctor explain to each one in turn the complexities of mama's operation, or is he heartless to ask the family to designate a representative to deal with him? Very often the most junior person on the complicated hospital treatment team, the medical student, is the one who spends the most time with families. This is partly because he wishes to learn from them, and partly because no one else has any *time* for them.

It is usually during the third and fourth year that students learn the role families play in patient care, and make the first steps, good or bad, toward dealing with them. Many studies and much anecdotal evidence show that dealing with families is a major unresolved source of concern and challenge for the medical profession. That is one reason that I have dwelled on it at length. Many people feel that the job is not being done as well as it should be. I try not to make any value judgments here, and neither should you, for no facile or one-sided accusations or responses are appropriate. This issue will be of particular interest to those of you who were influenced to choose medicine because of the quality of medical care given to members of your family when you were younger, and the impressions it left.

It may seem strange, but I think another major area of difficulty for students is coming to terms not only with disease, patients, and families, but *with treatment itself*. This can be a dilemma for people coming onto the wards, particularly if treatment is especially mutilating, destructive, questionable, risky, or simply frightening to behold and perform. (This applies equally to diagnostic procedures, which may or may not be directly therapeutic.) Because the state of the art is such that we cannot cure everything with a pill, bandage, or diet, we *do* resort to cutting people, cauterizing them, shocking them, debriding their avulsed and contaminated wounds, and strapping them into contraptions and appliances that restrict their every motion. Some patients are so intubated, tied down, hooked up, sandbagged, machine-connected, and needled, they have lost all control over not only voluntary, but involuntary functions of life.

Is it any wonder that a sensitive individual may have trouble confronting what he has to do to "help" the patient? Many of our treatment methods are so incomplete, inadequate, unsatisfactory, temporary, palliative, and based on empirical reasoning, our desires for more positive procedures are frustrated, and our scientific selves are offended. We have guilt when ugly side effects and unpleasant consequences occur, no matter how prepared we are for them in a statistical sense. We also know the "outside world" will misinterpret our attempts to help, and will blame us personally for whatever goes wrong. Who was it who started that god-doctor myth, and why don't they forget it at a time like this? Not only are *we* dissatisfied with our treatments, society is, too, and when they are sufficiently upset or misguided, they sue us for malpractice!

The discomfort response need not be triggered only by hot social issues, such as mastectomy or electric shock. It can be experienced by simple and relatively unheroic orders. For example, it was no picnic putting people on Sippy diets for gastric ulcers, for they were forced to down huge amounts of milk and cream and stuff that tasted like cardboard. Would *you* want to be subjected to such an awful menu for weeks at a time, even with the pain of an ulcer? And then suddenly someone decides that it is not very efficacious, anyway, and the diet goes out of style. Things like that do happen!

I recall being repelled by electro-convulsive therapy for catatonic and depressed patients while working in a state mental hospital. (This treatment has gotten a bad press, because it engenders similar feelings in many people.) But I also saw it work, almost miraculously, and we had nothing else that worked better. What do you do when you know you may damage a patient, but want to help and have no other choice? Along the same lines, there has been resistance on the part of the public and medical students alike to the "chemical straitjacketing" of schizophrenic patients by large doses of the major tranquilizers, but who remembers the "good old days" when thousands of patients screamed and shrieked under the torment of their persecutory fantasies, and we had little to give them? No, it is not pleasant to make "zombies" of your patients, but is it better for them to throw themselves out of windows to escape the dread voices that tell them to kill themselves because they are so wicked?

Some people have trouble even "sticking" patients for routine bloods. When they fail once, twice, or even three times, their hands start to sweat. In places where it's not the custom for nurses to be trained to come around to start IV drips, the interns make pacts with themselves that if they can't "get the vein" by the third stick, they'll call in a classmate to do it. (Some nights you just can't get it together.)

It is customary to have some anticipatory dread about the first days in surgery. Students wonder what it feels like to draw a knife across a pale vulnerable belly, one that is going up and down because its owner is *breathing* (unlike the first patient of freshman days). Usually they're so busy trying to see the operation (there's a lot of competition for limited belly space), or trying to stop the immediate bleeding, they don't have time for anything else. Most surgeons let the third-year students cut the knots.

Like everything else, experience brings philosophical resolution of many worries about prescribing certain therapies. A good doctor will never consider the issue permanently closed, but will evaluate new and old treatments in light of current knowledge. And, of course, he will never confuse reluctance to use a treatment with errors in *using* that treatment. It goes almost without saying that proper choices, dosages, time frames, and therapeutic alternatives are all part of the technical material physicians must master as they treat patients. Also remember that as the student becomes more proficient at performing certain tricky procedures, he becomes more at ease with them. This has its negative side in that he may forget that the patient is as much a novice at handling heroic treatments as *he* once was.

There is a major challenge that accompanies the understanding of disease and the interaction with the individual patient and his or her family. This involves *the ability to transcend one's background*, upbringing, personal beliefs, value systems, and other cultural trappings in order to be able to help patients and families who approach the world in an entirely different way. If it is possible for you to take one or two courses in sociology (not just that boring introductory course) or, even better, cultural anthropology when in college, please do so. It will help sensitize you to the problems people can get into when they don't understand the world from which the other party comes, and don't realize the importance of doing so. So many beliefs are deeply ingrained in us, particularly if we are the "majority culture" in this country, that are simply not shared by some of our patients; and if we try to impose our own standards on them, we end up with noncompliance, personal frustration, sicker patients, hostile interactions, and eventually "burn out," a phenomenon we'll discuss later. Besides, as hateful as the thought is to us, we might actually be *wrong*. Or, even if we are "right," if it is not "right" for the patient, it is still "wrong." Perhaps (liberating thought) there is no right *or* wrong.

"Culture conflicts" with patients are rife in the big cities of our country, where student doctors tear their hair over the parental use of garlic instead of penicillin for childhood bronchitis. They deplore giving coffee to kids, salty ethnic foods to pregnant ladies with swollen ankles, and amulets to infants who should be kept in sterile environments. All they end up with is alopecia (baldness).

In addition to culture conflicts with patients, there may be more with authority figures, professors, and attending physicians on the wards who have been raised in a different time and with different attitudes and mores. Often, student-teacher conflicts are centered around the management of patients who present a *third* standard of what may be right. For example, consider the case of a middle-aged woman with a husband, three kids, a full-time job, no house-hold help, and a marginal income and savings account. Her mother, a lovely lady from the Caribbean Islands, has been taken ill with a chronic disease and requires heavy nursing care for a prolonged period of time. The patient, raised to honor her parent and provide for her in her old age no matter what the personal cost, will be stressed to the breaking point if she fulfills her sense of obligation. There is little doubt that her present responsibilities, so carefully juggled, will all start to suffer, and her diabetes will probably get out of control again. (Since she'll be sleeping in the bathtub with water dripping on her head, she'll probably get pneumonia, too.)

The attending physician in this case is a no-nonsense sort whose parents died in an accident when he was nineteen. He feels that the patient's top priority should be to take care of herself, so that she doesn't end up in his emergency room in diabetic coma complicated by pneumonia. He believes strongly in the physician as decision maker and order giver, and has little conflict about telling the patient that if she knows what's good for her, she'll put the old lady in a nursing home. He will consider his duties discharged if he refers his patient to a good social worker who will help her find a reputable home that is close to her house and serves Spanish food.

The medical student, however, brings a different tradition and memory bank to the situation. He remembers what his mother went through when his father's sister broke her hip and came to live with them for three months. But he also remembers how his mother cried for months because her mother had cancer and she lived too far away to be able to go home to help. The entire burden of care had fallen on his uncle, whose wife hadn't been too helpful in the situation. He realizes what a toll *not* discharging one's self-perceived duties can take on an illness. Who's to say that the diabetes won't get worse with the old mama in a nursing home?

The patient's husband, whose parents were in show business and divorced when he was two, pretty much raised himself on the streets. He has trouble understanding a cultural sense of indebtedness, and sees only the reality of the situation. His predictable, utilitarian response is to let the old lady fend for herself. She has neighbors, doesn't she? What do other old people do who *don't* have children?

Clearly there are many attitudes and potential resolutions for this very common situation. The student must learn to evaluate his own attitudes, the patient's and family's opinions, and the thoughts of others involved in the treatment. Does he share the attending physician's belief in unilateral decision making, or does he consider it authoritarian and paternalistic? Does he believe in a "team decision," or think the matter should be worked out solely by the woman after she has been given all the appropriate medical facts for her situation? Is he influencing the patient to do what *he* would do if he were in her situation? Is he trying to get her to do what *he* believes is right (even if it may not be right for *her*, or he might not have the courage to do it himself)? Has he fulfilled his total obligation if he has dealt only with the "medical" facts, conveniently blocking out all the "social" facts over which he has no control (but which still complicate the patient's life)? Is it his place to advise the patient differently from his superior officer, or should he be a "team player"? You understand by now how important these decisions are.

Students quickly learn which attending physicians, senior residents, and other supervisors share or do not share their cultural backgrounds. There are some with whom they are in constant conflict. There are others who share their prejudices and do not help them to grow and reach beyond their own narrow background, probably because they were never able to do it themselves. The struggles between students and faculty center around ethical and cultural issues that are very familiar to you, as you have been through many with your teachers and parents. They are issues of "lying" to the patient, being a "double agent" who purports to serve both the patient and his employer at the same time, and "withholding" information because the doctor is "too busy to talk."

The list is quite long, and we will not tackle it now. Just be aware that becoming a clinical student means having your value systems challenged, shaken to the core, dumped overboard, or doubly reinforced. Every time you harangue a wife or child beater, every time you piously scold a self-neglecting patient, every time you moralize, preach, sneer, turn up a corner of your mouth, raise your voice, slip a chart to the bottom of the pile in punishment, or do any one of a number of such punitive actions, your culture is showing.

Because a medical student is not working with his patients and their families in isolation, adjustments will have to be made to the impersonal and complex *institution* that provides the climate and ambience for their activities. Often it is at variance with a student's early visions of a kindly doctor's office, where the nurses were known by name, and often were neighbors. The very buildings themselves can be intimidating at first. Consider that students train only in major medical centers, complexes large and prestigious enough to support an expensive school of medicine. Or they may work in ancillary institutions capable of accepting students through an affiliation agreement, by virtue of quality or proximity. Plunged into a generally frenetic environment (unless lucky enough to be assigned to a small community hospital), the new doctors often feel like aliens in clinic-land. Accustomed to honoring the ABSOLUTELY NO ADMITTANCE signs they remember from childhood visits to the hospital, they now are granted access to operating suites, radiation departments, delivery rooms, and infectious-disease isolation units, where they feel like bulls in china shops for the first few days. (An inevitable sense of entitlement soon takes over, however!)

Once geographically familiar with strange wards, elevator banks that dump them in laundry rooms when they wanted the OR, and parking lots that are accessible only through forty-seven miles of underground corridors marked with colored arrows, they can settle down to "learning the system." In many ways, "the system" is far more important to learn than the practice of medicine, the understanding of disease, or the interaction with patients.

"The system" of medicine refers to the entire way in which it is structured in this country. It refers to the division of labor into specialties (probably around thirty in all), and the classification of sick people into "in-patients" and "out-patients" of health-care institutions such as the general and specialty hospitals, the clinics, the private doctors' offices, and ancillary institutions. It encompasses the chessboard of "other health professionals" and how they relate to the physicians on the scene. It deals with how medical care is financed and politically influenced on the "macro" and "micro" levels. Medical care organization can be dull to read about, and you'll pick up most of it as you go along, so I won't belabor it here.

Certain recurrent themes sharply influence a student's work, however, so let's mention them now. They reflect, for example, an unspoken system of care based upon ability to pay, diluted somewhat by the proliferation of "third-party payers," but still deeply rooted in tradition. You don't see too many of the old multibedded wards anymore, except in the oldest and poorest hospitals. These were huge, open spaces for charity patients, in which beds were lined up a few feet apart, giving the occupants virtually no visual or auditory privacy, and unlimited company, welcome and unwelcome. The sensitivity that medical students brought to this dismal scene varied. One of my classmates thought it was the most dehumanizing room he'd ever entered; another blithely responded that "these people" are used to sharing close quarters with others and would probably feel lonely in private or semiprivate rooms! By and large, most people think it is a good thing that they have been phased out. To understand the implications of this shift, you really should try doing some reading in the field of medical history. When you see pictures of starched and bustled nurses standing rigidly at attention when visiting physicians entered the long ward, you get a sense of how much medicine has changed.

Nevertheless, "classism" remains very much alive. I once worked in a hospital whose front door opened onto one of the city's most fashionable boulevards, just across from its great park. Uniformed doormen in epaulets stood there under a canopy to hail cabs for discharged patients. The *back* door, a full block away, opened onto the perimeter of the ghetto. This was the entrance used by the out-patients, who came to the clinics for free or government-assisted care. And *this* door was guarded by uniformed security officers with gun belts and small clubs. The contrast was mind-boggling.

For many students, the third year is the point in their education when they are made painfully aware of the poverty of many of their patients, and how it aggravates or even directly causes their illnesses. It has been demonstrated for over 150 years that living conditions and levels of affluence influence health far more than direct medical intervention, yet medical students are only able to offer their "lesser" alternative. On some level they suspect that it *is* a lesser alternative, although the ethos of the institution pressures them greatly to deny it.

There is no physician alive today who has not had to deal with this prototypical case: A four-year-old comes to the emergency room with acute pneumonia. It is controlled on penicillin, medicine's quintessential miracle drug. But now the child must go back out into the streets, returning to an apartment that is unheated, ice-cold water (if it runs at all), garbage and rats, crime, violence, poor supervision, inadequate diet—the works. There's no way that kid isn't going to come back sicker than ever, in two months or three. Has the doctor done his job by simply prescribing a drug? This dilemma is so standard, particularly in deteriorating neighborhoods, that all must come to grips with the fundamental philosophical questions it poses: What is the function of a physician? Where does his job begin and end? Where is his responsibility, and, ultimately, where does it end? Should he be involved in the social problems of his patients? Should he confine himself to what he knows and is trained to do? Should he offer only liaison and support to others designated to solve these problems? Few physicians are able to answer these questions to their satisfaction, although the good ones spend a lifetime trying.

Medical students, whose curious minds will carry them out into slum households (since unfortunately few medical school programs put their bodies out there any more), should be prepared for the frustrations of what they will find, and their relative inability to do too much about it at their level. They are clearly at risk of being utterly overwhelmed by the crush of patients and their problems, with no time to devote to them, no opportunity to get to know them as well as is necessary, and no expertise to offer in fighting often-doomed battles against the bureaucracy. They should also be prepared for having difficulties in understanding some patients, or even being able to identify with them when the cultural and language barriers are too great. This is often the greatest disillusionment of all.

Another significant attribute of "the system" is its fondness for certain kinds of illnesses, and certain kinds of patients. The system prefers exotic, rare, and tantalizing diseases rather than the common, predictable, and ultimately rather boring small illnesses that plague the lives of the masses. ("I think if I have to see another tonsillitis this morning, I'm going to go off my rocker!") We ought to call this phenomenon "anti-commonism"! Coupled with this is an enchantment with sudden, dramatic, acute illness, rather than the long-term, slow-change, incurable stuff with which many people grudgingly coexist. The above-mentioned illnesses tend to occur in younger people, who are considered more rewarding than the elderly and chronically ill who are not going to make dramatic improvements and send the doctor home glowing to his wife in the evening.

Students may be forgiven for quickly being "socialized" into sharing a physician's curiosity about the exotic, for technically it *is* the greatest intellectual challenge, and the reason he came to medical school. (Or was it because he wanted to help people?) Unfortunately, most patients suffer from perfectly ordinary disease, and when they are treated by someone who devalues it, they know and sense that they have disappointed their caretaker. They recognize that the best intellectual effort has not been brought to bear on making them feel better. Their doctor, or student, has begun to identify with those high-caste professors of earlier days who turned the masses over to their clerks, and saved their brains for the "good stuff." The more these attitudes are reinforced, the lesser the chances of the aged, the "crocks," the chronically ill to get the best medical care.

Since doctors are reflections of their society, they bring to their students and practices personal attitudes about race and sex that may conflict with the impenetrably egalitarian ideals of the Hippocratic Oath (if you omit slaves). This comes as a shock to students, although it certainly should not. Yes, there are some physicians who do not treat black female heads of households with the same manner they reserve for white males in the same tax-paying category. Medical students, particularly female students, have been doing a lot to counter these attitudes when they are displayed in teaching clinics.

Feminist women who have been active in the feminist women's

health movement state that women physicians are better to deal with than men, particularly the younger women. They are more given to sharing their expertise, without exaggerated concern for the possible negative effects, and less inclined to erect artificial barriers between physician and patient. This may be so.

It is particularly unfortunate that the student must encounter racial and sexual discrimination at a time when idealism is best able to express itself. In the case of sexual discrimination, an additional burden is put on the student who is learning to treat sexual disorders and treat sexual problems during the course of another illness. Male students, for example, simply cannot be expected to approach women for genital and rectal examinations without good teaching, helpful attitudes, and a chance to discuss their feelings. Where women are denigrated, insulted, put down, and dismissed, their chances of learning proper skills are markedly diminished. And if they don't watch out, they'll end up with an all-male practice—or a lot of women patients who really hate them.

The whole situation is best summed up in the "zebra/horse" dichotomy. An old medical axiom states that when one hears the sound of hoofbeats in the distance, it's wise to think of horses rather than zebras. It's our way of curbing the student who's conjuring up all kinds of rare diseases unnecessarily. We're saying, "Don't always think of the rare and exotic; think what statistically the disease is most likely to be." But the double message and unwritten rule is simply that he who finds the most zebras climbs highest in the medical jungle. So zebras it continues to be. Someday, they will actually dedicate a new medical institution entitled "The Hospital of the Black and White Striped Horse." Or perhaps they will drop that high-falutin' language and simply call it "The Zebra Medical Center." It will be well named.

In the search for rare equines, a broad and extensive net must be cast. In hospitals, this translates into very expensive "work-ups." A complete work-up involves sending many tubes of blood to the lab for diagnostic evaluation, X-rays, scans, collection of body fluids and sections for study, calling in consultants to help with the evaluation, and so on. If you have not seen an itemized hospital bill following a fairly complete diagnostic work-up, you have not tasted high finance. These bills make current interest rates look like Monopoly money. Please ask the administrator of your local hospital to give you access to some blind sample hospital statements. It's a necessary part of your education.

Students, again, are caught in the squeeze more than most. One day an attending physician will give it to them for having worked up the patient too extensively, thereby running up the bill. The next day they'll get balled out for failing to get a serum transaminase on Mr. Jones. They can't win!

The system expresses itself dramatically in the social environment it creates. A clinical student tends to get dropped into this environment like a nut dropped onto the rocks by a high-flying bird of prey who can't break it open with his beak. It is a very structured, hierarchical, conservative, and tradition-bound environment. In it, the student is seen as both the crown prince and precious repository for all knowledge of past and future generations, and the lowly apprentice who has to be carefully supervised lest he stir the wrong pot or spill the porridge all over his smock. Unsure what their place is in the grand scheme of things, students are forever in terror that they have undertaken too much or been too passive in performing their duties. Few hospitals are shored up to help students with their anxiety. The needs of the patient come first, and students are left to deal with their uncertainties and professional maturation as best they can.

Students learn from the intern and resident (and the nurses), even more than from senior physicians, primarily because they work most closely with them and are but a few years behind them in training. But they soon become aware of all hospital personnel, and their place in the order of things. They also tune in to the physical plant, for treatment depends upon how well it functions. When the boiler breaks and patients and staff alike freeze, the students know it. They know when linens don't make it back from the laundry, when night floats don't show, when the diet kitchen runs amuck, when a classmate makes an idiot of himself on rounds. They know when a patient dies under a cloud, when a service has had a budget cut over the protests of the director (not that it did him any good!), when the record room is behind on charts, and when key equipment is on the fritz. They know when a major researcher has had a feud with a rival, when a labor union is threatening the wildcat strike to end all wildcat strikes, when a story appeared in the local newspaper that made heads roll down every corridor in the institution.

Clinical students are part of the place. In some cases, they are uninvolved bystanders with no direct responsibility except to learn. In others, they may have been the unwitting trigger point. From the plunge onto those rocks, however, they gain experience, learn techniques, develop attitudes, grow as physicians, and become eligible for promotion.

The junior and senior years are exciting, exhilarating, scary, wonderful, exhausting, but, above all, real. I really hope you are getting a picture of what the new life is like. It is a time when students become a part of the profession in every sense. It is a time when they begin to realize just what kind of doctors they are going to become. It is a time of using role models, exploring specialties, gaining confidence, correcting mistakes, and gaining a broad base of experience. By the time the fourth year begins, the student doctor is very much a doctor, indeed. Never mind that he still has classes to attend, exams to take, courses to pass, and academic considerations to contend with. His final year will be primarily "electives," and after that, graduation!

We will be talking more about the senior year (and graduation) in the next chapter, for in spirit and outlook it is more closely allied to the internship year than those that preceded it. Keenly aware that a few words of mumbo-jumbo on rapidly approaching Graduation Day may confer instant doctorhood, but not instant competence, the student hovers on the brink of the last open space before his final goal has been attained. Close on the horizon, he sees the years of post-graduation training that will follow as the night the day (and possibly the next night, too!). Let's have a look at what is in store.

Getting Experience: Internship and Residency

9.

Are
You a Doctor
or a House Officer?

The year that precedes postgraduate training is generally spent polishing skills, building confidence, and breathing a little on electives. Schools are now quite generous in permitting their students to travel and work in other institutions. (They are *so* generous, sometimes I wonder if they aren't doing a little dumping.) Fourth-year students now can do research projects, have intensive clinical experiences in interesting specialties, do a tutorial, write a survey paper, study abroad, or even become involved in a health-related social or political project in community health.

The loose structure of the senior year also enables them to make plans for their postgraduate training, which is of great importance in determining their future careers. Some students know by now which area of medicine most appeals to them; others sweat because they haven't made up their minds and know that their ambivalence and uncertainty are working against them. By and large, this is true, because the system is geared to early decision and commitment. The desire to obtain a good internship and residency can force some students into premature decisions that they may regret at some point in the future.

The seniors in any given year spend a good chunk of the fall visiting hospitals to inspect their graduate training facilities, talk to incumbent house staff, and assess their chance of acceptance (significantly enhanced if they have done an outstanding undergraduate elective there). They then trust their fates to the Great Computer that matches hospitals with programs to offer, with students who want to undertake them. When the Giant Button is pushed one day in March, the bulletin board of every school in the country is plastered with huge sheets listing who's been accepted where. Lucky are those who have gotten their first choice, for many will have to be satisfied with a hospital they ranked farther down the list because of its location, pay scale, on-call schedule, or reputation. A few don't match at all, due to some unforeseen circumstance, and they have to scrounge outside the "matching" system for a place to continue their education.

The choice of a good internship and, subsequently, a residency in a particular specialty is really critical, for the postgraduate training scene is one that is easily turned sour. Graduate doctors learn their trade by working in a hospital that offers them a good mix of patient care, formal or informal academic teaching, and the opportunity, perhaps, to do a little research. In hospitals where service requirements are unusually high (such as the municipal and county hospitals rich in poor patients without private physicians or non-academically affiliated community hospitals), the intern may be caught up in an unpleasant and exhausting situation where he is working a hundred hours a week doing routine chores. He loses the opportunity to see interesting patients, or read about them when he does. It is of paramount importance that a graduating student land a position in a medical center that has a superb attending staff, recognizes and honors its commitments to its house staff, and makes their time worthwhile.

As you'd expect, the best hospitals want the best graduates. It is for this reason that students cannot totally drop their preoccupation with grades once they get into medical school. At the present time, some schools have been experimenting with the "pass-fail" grading system, in the hope that competition would be kept down to a dull roar. But the modification, "pass with honors," has upset the whole applecart, for students with "honors" became the new elite for hospital scouts. A letter in a recent issue of *The New England Journal of Medicine* offered the results of an informal survey of sixty-one competitive, in fact, highly rated hospitals, by researchers at the University of Connecticut. They found that residency directors tended to favor graduates of standard grading programs, where at least they knew what they were getting. I suspect that "pass-fail" may not last for this reason.

Choosing the right specialty, as mentioned above, is a serious hurdle for the senior student. In the old days, most graduating physicians did a one-year "rotating" internship (where they got a sample of everything), then immediately went out into general practice. The three- to five-year residencies in the hospitals went to those who had the time, money, and dedication to become specialists. When changing times and circumstances reversed this trend, the country found itself with a sharp drop in generalists, and a predominance of physicians who had become the ultimate authority on the right nostril or the left eyelid. Once again the pendulum is swinging back, and just in time for you. You now have your choice of many specialities, and general practice as well, the latter being updated to include a hospital residency, an increased emphasis on didactic training, and even certification by the new Board of Family Medicine. It is now virtually unheard of for a student to walk right out of an internship (necessary for a state license) without at least considering one or more years of postgraduate training.

Choosing the right specialty is difficult because our computerized society forces students to make a lifetime decision before they have even completed their fourth year of medical school. Many have not yet rotated through some of the services that might have proved to be just the field they would have wanted. Luck, chance, calculated risk, and intuition are the basic factors in such cases. That they are not foolproof is evidenced by the large number of physicians who drop out of residencies and relocate elsewhere; or even switch specialties in mid-career, returning for a second residency at a time that represents a real financial hardship.

One would have to summarize the basic challenges of the senior year as the following: choosing an appropriate specialty, obtaining a good internship and residency in that field, and learning as much as possible before graduation. Sometimes, having to do all three at once seems utterly impossible, but by April, with only six weeks to go to finals and graduation, most students have made their peace with their decisions and can look forward to the next major phase of their education with a certain equanimity.

The final days of medical school resemble the last days before the birth of a baby. Nobody rocks the boat, and the time spent waiting for the big event is full of delightful trivia. Students begin slipping away weekends to leave APARTMENT WANTED notes on the bulletin boards of Laundromats, and compose elaborate APART-MENT FOR RENT signs to dispose of the old ones. Some students begin ordering graduation announcements from the printer and selling books they, erroneously, think they'll never have to use again to underclassmen whose ordeal is not yet over.

Many institutions will schedule special events in recognition of the forthcoming "rite of passage." In my school, we had a celebratory Hundred Day Dinner, which was a formal banquet for students, spouses, and faculty, at which the great countdown to graduation began. Those hundred days were spent getting used to the realization that student days would soon be gone forever. Before we knew it, we suddenly found ourselves capped and gowned, and surrounded by a sea of professors dressed in the velvet robes and tassled mortarboards of close to a hundred universities.

Graduation Day is probably the most momentous occasion in a student's life, and the one whose memory he brings green to his internship. I am writing this at the time the American hostages have returned from Iran to their familial reunions at West Point, and the aura of incredulous relief and happiness reminds me very much of the feelings of a medical-school graduate the morning the black gown is donned with its three doctoral stripes on the sleeve.

Of the three graduations I remember best, one was my friend's and one was my own. Although in different cities, and at different times, they were both characterized by that same quality: a giddy, infectious, unrestrained joyousness. If ever you want a real high, sneak in the back doors at a medical-school graduation. You'll see grown people bursting with pride, weeping with happiness, hugging complete strangers, and posing with their doctor children under every tree.

At my friend's graduation, parents were asked to stand for a round of applause from grateful students. Then spouses were asked to stand for a cheer from their doctor partners. Even grandparents got a chance to throw kisses. But what brought the house down was a final round of cheers when infants and toddlers were hoisted aloft to be thanked for all those hours of good behavior while mommy and daddy did their thing.

I was the first to walk down the aisle at my graduation, because my name began with a B. My knees were knocking when I walked across the stage to shake the dean's hand, receive my diploma, and have the green velvet-lined doctoral hood slung around my neck. I was sure she was going to change her mind and make me go back for some remedial work. But she sent me off the stage to be a doctor. It was the most exciting moment of my life until the day, many years later, when the rabbi looked up impatiently at the wedding guests assembled in my living room and said, "OK, folks, let's get this show on the road."

I feel sorry for those who finished medical school during the revolutionary periods of the past few years and felt compelled to receive their diplomas in the mail. It's a lot like getting married at City Hall; you're still married, but your moment of truth has never been publicly confronted and assimilated. So many fears, hopes, emotions, feelings are bound up in Graduation Day, and come welling out in a great social catharsis!

❖   ❖   ❖

The life of an intern is an exhausting, exhilarating, crazy, terrifying, fulfilling one. (Do those words sound familiar?) The intern
is plunged into a continuous, almost nonstop treadmill of sick people in various stages of work-up, treatment, convalescence, or
even stagnation and neglect. At times he may remember those
days when he didn't get to see any patients as belonging to his remote past. Most of the time, he's too tired for anything but the job
at hand.

It's important to understand very well the backdrop of *fatigue
and sleeplessness* against which most interns have to function. For
many, only the fun of the work and the dedication to its meaning
shield against the all-pervasive desire to go to sleep and stay that
way for a long time. Hospitals vary in their "on-call" schedules,
most requiring their interns to work every second or third night
and every second or third weekend, in addition to their five-and-
a-half-day, fifty-five-hour work week. This means arrival on the
floor at about seven or eight in the morning and working through
to six or seven the evening of the *following* night if one has been
on call; or until six or seven the same night if one is "off." (Surgeons tend to work longer hours.) If one works the weekend, it
means showing up on a Saturday morning and going home Monday evening. Although the intern is provided with a room to sleep
in during his nights on call, he is awakened for every call on his
service, and it is seldom that he sleeps uninterruptedly. It is not
unusual for the intern to work through the night with no break at
all, or with only catnaps of an hour or two at a stretch. On a busy
weekend, the intern can work for up to sixty hours without
sleep! He becomes accustomed to seeing fresh teams of nurses reporting every eight hours, over and over, while he is still starting
IVs and doing admission physicals. On a weekend, he can even
see Nurse Jones come in in the morning, put in her eight hours, go
home for dinner and a good night's sleep, and come back to work
the next day, three times running, during which hours he has not
had time for more than a quick shower to refresh!

It is important for you to try to imagine this state of sleep deprivation, and place yourself in it, for it pervades the intern's being. Even those who are on an every-third-night call schedule are only slightly better off. Since the workdays require a great deal of running around, climbing flights of stairs two at a time, dashing to lab and X-ray, and racketing all around a fairly large institution, you can see how important it is for the intern to be a healthy specimen.

Although my internship year was the most exciting, stimulating, and rewarding year of my life, I do remember experiencing this sleep-starved syndrome. There were days when I would make rounds and see my own handwriting on a chart, ordering medications for a patient from the previous night, and I would have no recollection of ever having been there at all! Often I functioned as a complete zombie, performing the most intricate manipulations on patients with my eyes half closed and my body temperature down several degrees to its nocturnal level. Chilled, zonked, headachey, muscle-bound, and only half awake, I would take call after call, passing catheters, restarting IVs, catching babies, and evaluating passing episodes of nausea, vomiting, diarrhea, incontinence, and hallucinations. I even wrote back-to-sleep orders for patients whose sleeplessness seemed downright blasphemy to an intern who would have pushed the patient right out of bed to grab it for herself.

Every doctor can tell you the bizarre things that happened to him as a result of fatigue. For example, I remember once driving home in the afternoon rush hour on one of Philadelphia's busiest highways. My fan belt broke in the middle of the road, and I pulled over on the median to await help. Ordinarily, I would have found it nerve-wracking to be stranded in the middle of six lanes of cars speeding by like whizzing bullets, but on this occasion I'd been up for several nights. I fell dead asleep over the wheel, awakening only when a cop starting pounding on my window with a look on his face that said, "You crazy lady, how could you possibly fall asleep at a time like this?" (This was before drugs.) By the time I got home I was really out of it. I went to wash my hands before falling asleep, and stood there for about five minutes vainly trying to get a lather. I then discovered that I'd been vigorously massaging a tube of toothpaste!

No one wants to think that house staff responsible for human lives are making fatal errors because they're too zonked to think. (Jaded interns are tempted to say, "Who needs to think?") In fact, researchers periodically come up with studies that attempt to prove that this is actually happening. Still, it is amazing how efficiently even exhausted people can perform, and the miracle is that more damage doesn't take place.

Closely allied to an intern's fatigue is the overwhelming threat of being inundated by *scutwork*, even in the best of training programs. The house officer can spend only a small portion of his time visiting, examining, and treating patients. Even less can be spent in conference or the library. The remainder is spent on the firing line of the war between bureaucracy and patient care. At the risk of making you as bored as the intern, I'll discuss just a few of the noninspirational chores with which the poor soul gets saddled.

The intern spends his life writing—longhand, at that. Amazing as it sounds, few hospitals offer the kind of dictating equipment for routine notes that is generally afforded the most menial clerk on Madison Avenue. The intern must write detailed histories and physicals on the patient's chart, and add daily progress notes. These include pre-op notes, operative notes, post-op notes, delivery notes, and find-something-to-say notes, even when the patient's status is completely unchanged. Hospitals demand these notes, for they are necessary for accreditation and to protect the institution against lawsuits. Most interns get so far behind on their charts, they are in constant trouble with the record room. Recently, enterprising hospital administrators with hearts of ice have taken to withholding the offender's paycheck until he has scribbled himself back into good graces. This was recently tested in the courts and found to be illegal, so some other petty vengeance will probably be exacted from the intern's hide.

House officers get stuck with explaining preoperative procedures to patients who are notoriously unable to remember ever having heard one word of the discourse, and to relatives who are unable to retain the information until they have heard it at least three times. They must then get patients and/or their legal guardians to sign "consent" forms, which is often about as easy as getting someone to sign for a vacation cruise to Devil's Island.

Since interns are responsible for ordering, tracking, and sitting on top of their patients' lab work, and since a great deal of it is ordered, much time is spent in follow-up. In hospitals where the lab is understaffed, poorly functioning, or deficient, the intern finds himself becoming clerk, secretary, messenger, or often even lab tech himself. On nights and weekends, he'll do a lot of the lab work himself, desperately staining blood smears and peering at them with his one good eye through a microscope that should have been retired after World War II.

Interns desperate to get their patients to X-ray have been known to push the stretchers themselves, rather than go through the hassle of tracking, finding, cajoling, stealing, or blackmailing an orderly into doing the job for which he was hired.

Interns are often mistaken for other people in the hospital and asked to perform duties that are not strictly theirs. If they have a kind heart and a team spirit, they'll often comply. Women physicians, especially, get hauled into patients' rooms to remove and empty bedpans, since all women in white have to be nurses. They hoist patients up onto operating tables, cart them off into wheelchairs, and have been known to drop things off on the third floor for nurses who are even more overwhelmed than they are.

Drawing blood is both a diagnostic and therapeutic procedure, so interns have to become very proficient at entering veins. When I was an intern, only doctors were allowed to pounce on a patient with a needle, but nowadays nurses are trained especially for the purpose, and usually do the job with more finesse and loving care than any house officer. Their presence has eased the intern's job, in that this scutwork needs to be performed less often, but it makes it harder when the nurses aren't around, for the skill is not as well developed. When a phlebotomist is on night call, an intern gets more sleep. And he gets spoiled rotten.

Veins have to be entered not only to get blood to send to the lab, but to instill intravenous infusions of blood and sugar water with medications. These infusions have a nasty way of clogging up in the middle of the night, and must be flushed out or restarted in another vein. Some patients run out of easily accessible veins, necessitating a more complicated entry to the venous system. There is a fine line between therapeutic procedure and scutwork, and the vein is surely it.

Patients often require a number of minor procedures to aid their treatment, convalescence, or state of well-being. It is the intern who decides whether this activity constitutes doctoring or scutwork. Among these procedures I'd include passing catheters into urinary bladders to facilitate the passage of urine; aspirating mucus-clogged breathing passages through suction machines; extensive changing of dressings for large body-surface wounds; and so forth. In hospitals where interns are at a premium, there is a greater tendency to offer these duties to nurses, these duties being hastily redefined as not necessitating a physician's skill. Young doctors who have transferred from hospitals that permit the nurses greater latitude in direct care of this sort can get very annoyed when they find themselves in an institution that arbitrarily has decided that no one but the doctor may perform a specific procedure.

There are times when even an incontrovertibly therapeutic act is viewed as scutwork. The intern, particularly the intern on call at night, is called upon to write orders for patients whose physicians have gone home for the day. Sometimes an emergency develops, more often it is due only to carelessness that the patient is left without written orders for constipation, pain, sleeplessness, diarrhea, and the like. The intern is often called in the middle of the night to write for an immediate dose of painkiller or soporific, when it all could and should have been handled earlier by the physician whose task it was. Interns hate to be called for dumb reasons, and most nurses understand that it is not because they are unfeeling, heartless people, but because they need the sleep more than the patients do.

Discharge paperwork is the curse of the intern's existence, and it is because of environmental and circumstantial factors over which he has no control. The forms that must be filled out to get a patient onto Medicaid, Medicare, or some other third-party payer can be attended to only in part by the social worker—and not all hospitals use them. The medical part of the form must be filled in by a doctor, and always the low doctor on the totem pole. An intern's greatest nightmare is trying to transfer an elderly, sick, borderline senile patient to whatever institution will take him. Nursing homes, extended-care facilities, health-related facilities, domiciliary-care facilities, old-age homes are all tapped in a frantic attempt to get the patient out of a valuable hospital bed and into a less expensive, more appropriate facility.

Matching the patient with the requirements of the various institutions, and then matching again according to ability to pay or the possibility of insurance coverage, is a hideous task for doctor and social worker alike, given the inadequacy of available beds outside and the pressures to discharge the patient inside. When patients can't return to their own homes, or to those of their children, each elderly person becomes a major placement challenge. Since it is such an unpleasant task, there is a tendency to push it off until just before the patient is ready to leave, when in fact it is best started the day the patient first comes to the hospital. But another problem is the lability of such patients, whose condition changes from one day to the next, and for whom advance planning is extremely difficult. In the last analysis, the intern is stuck with all the human misery, and paperwork, the phone calls, the explanatory conversations, and often the raw investigative work as well. Sick, elderly patients, for whom the intern should feel the most compassion, engender the most scutwork. It affects the relationship.

An intern intent on avoiding scutwork at all costs (and there is a distinction between necessary scutwork and unnecessary scutwork) early learns to identify those patients who have I CAUSE SCUTWORK branded in invisible letters on their foreheads. The elderly are only one example. Another group of patients includes all those admitted through the emergency room for some terrible, acute condition that the intern knows very well will clear up in a day or two under intensive treatment, but who will lie around on the floor taking up a valuable bed for weeks and weeks because of a placement problem.

Placement problems who generate scutwork include alcoholics who are bleeding and sick and must be stabilized, but who then cannot be discharged, for sending them out into the streets with no shelter runs the risk of a lawsuit for the hospital. They include borderline welfare cases where no one is sure who is going to pay the bill, or if it will be paid at all. They include anyone from a rooming house or boarding home where the landlady will not guarantee keeping a patient's room for him until he returns from the hospital. They include transfers from nursing homes, patients who have developed an acute episode of something on top of their underlying disease and may not be reaccepted back into the home when the hospital stay is concluded. Placement problems mean paperwork, heartache, frustration, countless phone calls and letters, conferences with other health-care team members, and a notorious feeling of no-win. When an intern meets a patient whose forehead says I CAUSE SCUTWORK, his own forehead lights up with I CAN'T WIN.

Fatigue and scutwork cause major challenges to the new physician, but they are not the only ones. A third that rates high on the list of items for you to think about now are *status problems*. I'm not referring here to just being the low man on the four-year-cycle totem pole that was discussed back in Chapter Three. I mean that there are still real identity problems for house staff that cause gnawing resentments and sap some of their energies if exaggerated by political agitation.

Since the beginnings of modern medicine, no one has been able to decide once and for all whether a house officer is a student or a worker. Clearly there are elements of both service and education in his daily routine, but how much of each? When I was an intern, less than twenty years ago, we considered ourselves students and were thrilled when our monthly wage was raised from one hundred dollars a month to one hundred and fifty. After all, we got free room, board, and uniforms, and our predecessors had earned exactly zero during their three- to five-year stint. And they had worked longer hours than we! Today there is more of a tendency to think of the intern as an employee of the hospital, there to learn while he gives service, and the going wage is around sixteen thousand dollars a year, and rising every June.

There are reality implications in whether an intern is considered a student or a worker. For years there's been an ongoing dispute between the IRS, which has tended to view house staff as workers and therefore liable to pay income tax on their earnings, and the National Labor Relations Board, which has tended to view them as students and their earnings as honoraria, or fellowships, which are partially exempt from the clutches of the government.

If a house officer sees himself as a worker, he will invariably be displeased with his wages and compare his earnings with those of executive secretaries, computer programmers, and others who make more money than he does after eight years of higher education. He will be bitter and militant and walk around feeling constantly ripped off. On the other hand, if he views himself primarily as a student who is learning in a field-site placement, he will be constantly resentful that so many service demands are made upon him, leaving him no time, energy, or opportunity to learn, which is why he came in the first place. The house officer is up against a real no-win situation again, and this one gets him where he lives—in the pocketbook and in the intellect.

Unable to resolve this dilemma, because there really *is* no possible resolution, a number have embarked on political activity to enforce either one demand or the other. It is my personal bias that this flurry of activity is really a diversionary maneuver that helps relieve the pain of the identity crisis. Unable to identify a clear enemy and a clear position, and because they are too fair to be one-sided, house staff seize upon one issue or the other and try to resolve it directly. The movement toward unionization of house staff is strong in this country, and there has been a good deal of organizing around house staff associations in various hospitals. Attending physicians (who feel that if unionization of house staff is imminent, can their own unionization be far behind) get very politicized and stirred up over the issue. In the background lurks the specter of national health insurance and a socialized system. So in today's world, everything gets blown out of proportion. Those of you interested in hot issues in medicine today should look with interest on this aspect of an intern's life. How would *you* feel?

Part of this problem comes back to the intern's keen awareness of how much he has to learn, and how many superior officers are watching over his work, he who is supposed to be an autonomous professional and who has put in so much time getting where he is. He's generally dissatisfied with his role in the hierarchy, and he has every reason to be, particularly when his first- or second-year resident is not as sharp or capable as he is, but is awarded more money, status, and authority.

I'm thinking of one specific example of this dissatisfaction—the house officer's role in the medical research that is so critical to the advancement of scientific knowledge, and the professional rise of the young scientist who undertakes it. Medical students and junior house officers are sometimes given the opportunity to work with a senior scientist, often a departmental chief and/or a top name in the field. Often these young researchers contribute more than routine service, such as injecting rats or pulling agar plates out of the incubator at 6:00 A.M. Sometimes they are intimately involved with the research design and the intellectual basis of the experiment itself. Yet, according to protocol, when the papers reporting the results of the experiments are published (let us hope in prestigious journals), the senior author is generally the top man, and the fellow who did most, if not all, of the actual work is listed in small print down at the end of the line. A generous and fair chief will give credit where it is due, and it is not unheard of for a top person to let the intern place his name first on the paper. Others are not so scrupulous, and intellectual rip-offs in the world of research and big-money grants take place every day of the year.

When inequities are perceived, the intern can end up feeling resentful, and that's all the good it will do him. There's nothing he can do or say, for he is an unknown, and the senior scientist has money, prestige, and a reputation (which the intern is sure was earned on the backs of generations of innocents like himself). The ethics of research relationships need to be studied carefully in the future, for reasons more important than merely the status-seeking of interns.

A bad resident can make an intern's life utterly miserable, just as a good medical student can sweeten it with scientific curiosity and an eagerness to learn. A bad resident can send in unflattering evaluations that can seriously hamper an intern's future career, if corroborated by similar remarks from attending physicians. Fortunately, interns now have an opportunity to review their folders and refute, if necessary, remarks that have been made about them that they feel are unfair, erroneous, or based on inadequate information. House officers may now be paid as employees, but in the evaluation process, they still feel very much like students.

Another source of irritation for many, which is status connected, is their position as recipients of student loans that now must be renegotiated or paid back at this inopportune time. There is nothing like the pressure of a creditor to make an insecure person feel even more unworthy.

One way for the intern to extricate himself from status problems, including money issues, is to start planning a future outside the hospital. Most are unable to mobilize to do this until the third year of their residency, for more pressing daily issues take precedence. It is not until the cold, cruel world looms up after so many years in the institution that house officers start their futures.

The intern, of course, is not defenseless in handling the issues we have discussed here. One of his best defenses is that old gallows humor, the same grim laughter that got him through the anatomy lab, the wall-to-wall exams, and his first surgery. I recently came across a book that you probably should read called *The House Of God* by Dr. Samuel Shem. My first impulse was to discard it as just another trash novel exploiting sex and the single intern, but it came highly recommended from serious people, so I curled up with it one night. It was really a howl. Yes, it was utterly outrageous, exaggerated, filthy, cynical, and jaded, but oh, how funny! If you'll read it with a grain of salt, it will give you a good feeling for an intern's emotions while going through the meat grinder. I wouldn't be surprised if they made it into a movie. If so, it would probably be even funnier than *Hospital*, starring George C. Scott. I thought that one was a pretty good example of gallows humor, too!

Another good defense for the intern is a warm place to come home to. Naturally one would expect more house officers than medical students to be married, and an understanding spouse is probably the single greatest gift and stabilizing force a busy young doctor can have. A good partner makes the successes so much sweeter, and the failures much less painful. A house officer who is warmly loved and supported has half the battle won.

In the last analysis, it is important for the intern to be able to put all his gripes and pressures into one compartment, and just get down to the business of relating to his patients with as much curiosity, interest, and warmth as he can. And hospitals are full of rewarding, interesting, needy patients who do respond to therapy and are able to convey their gratitude and thanks to the intern who has helped them do it. (By the way, this includes all those "placement problems.") This may seem like a simple thing to do, but often it is not, particularly for the most idealistic of physicians. They did not anticipate all the things that would get in the way of their pure relationship with patients, and are confounded when forced to deal on compromise levels.

I have just finished reading a most moving excerpt from a new book entitled *The Bitter Pill* by Dr. Martin Lipp. It describes in vivid terms the gradual disillusionment of a young woman going through medical school and a residency in psychiatry. Described as a person who went into medicine identifying more closely with patients (having been one herself) than the medical establishment, she finds herself so overwhelmed with work she cannot be the empathic, relaxed, and caring physician she was so sure she was going to be. Faced with a long stretch on a drug ward, where she and everyone else are ripped off by manipulative young addicts, she becomes more guarded, more withdrawn, more in need of carving out a whole new ethic to keep her working for patients. In short, she has to become a realist, a compromiser, a pragmatist. Although she is suffering now, she will probably be the better for her journey through disillusionment. It was inevitable.

In trying to make one's peace with the discrepancies between the realities of what one wants to do for patients and what one *can* do for patients, friends, mentors, and support groups are invaluable. House officers who make unrealistic demands upon themselves, who blame themselves for failures that are system-based rather than personal mistakes, who are forced to turn away from one patient because another needs them more, who make a decision that is a clear error, who alienate patients or families unwittingly, all can find comfort from those most qualified to give it—people who know how hard they try, and how good they really are. I mentioned in an earlier chapter that student doctors have to take themselves apart and put themselves back together again before they go out on their own to practice. This is the process to which I was referring.

An intern just isn't *aware* unless he goes through some kind of burn-out period during the course of his training. With luck it will not last very long. People who have high ideals and heavy "rescue fantasies" may suffer feelings that they are not getting anywhere, not really affecting the lives or illnesses of their patients, not really of much use to anybody when they endure long periods of unrelieved stress. Sometimes this burn out takes the form of patient punishing and victim blaming. With a little help, house staff realize what they are doing and stop blaming people for not getting well, and punishing them for getting sick. It's a little bit like menopause. Some folks sail right through it and others get cramps and flashes. But sooner or later, it's over.

By the time a house officer has come to the end of his residency, his whole attitude toward patient care has changed tremendously. Suddenly aware that there is a "real world" out there, in which a personal niche must be found, a house officer goes through his final "weaning" process from the twelve years of training. He must decide on whether to take a salaried part- or full-time position in a hospital somewhere; whether or not to go out into private practice, and, if so, partnered or solo; whether or not to try a large group practice; or even whether or not to stay on in post-residency subspecialty training. He must decide whether or not to stay in a big city (which one?), or to fulfill the old dream to get out into a rural community where he's really needed. He's suddenly confronted with the fact that there will no longer be a whole built-in system to help him with decisions, cover his mistakes, prop him when he needs moral support. It's a time of anxiety and stress until it is all resolved.

The graduating resident is much like the graduating college senior and graduating medical student, clearly on the brink of a whole new life. Most of these people have passed serenely through their periods of "mini burn out," when all their work seemed futile and it was hard to get up in the morning. They have passed through many clinical challenges, and had enough successes with patients to feel that they are competent to go out on their own and make a difference. They have started to contact the people who can help them set up office, get stationery printed, do their more complicated income taxes, and find homes in new communities. They're on their way.

Many hospitals have banquets or small "graduation" ceremonies to honor their retiring house staff. They are generally more subdued, more businesslike, less well-attended than those of earlier days. (Those residents who will be sticking around, and maintaining an ongoing relationship with the hospital that trained them, are the most likely to come!) Often awards are given for the "best house officer" of the year. Despite all the cynicism, this person is usually the one who has been deemed by the staff to have had the most compassion, the best clinical skills, the greatest sense of fulfilling duties and obligations, and the best sense of humor to grace the above virtues. When the last day comes, on June 30 of every year, a whole cycle in medical education has been completed.

Private Thoughts for Special People

10.
When
You're a
Woman of Ambition . . .

In 1955, approximately 6 percent of the nation's physicians were women, a skimpy, imbedded statistic that had been unchanged for many years. About ten years ago, as a direct result of several key pieces of federal legislation dealing with discrimination in educational opportunities and health manpower appropriations, women started to come back into medicine in larger numbers. I say "come back" because, contrary to popular opinion, women in medicine were once thriving in this country, until their presence became a financial and social nuisance to men in the field. At that point, they were deliberately and systematically eradicated, almost as successfully as smallpox. For those of you interested in this abysmal historical note, consult a very enlightening book entitled *Doctors Wanted: No Women Need Apply* by Mary Roth Walsh, Ph.D.

It was with great fascination a few years ago that we "old-timers" watched the numbers of women increase to just about 30 percent of the entering classes. We happily predicted that someday the presence of these women would make itself known, and for the better, of course. Even when entry levels dropped back down to 25 percent, where they have since remained, we were optimis-

169

tic that the new personnel ratios would permit penetration of "feminine values" into the medical power structure, and effect humanization and softening of the approach to patients.

Many people shared my belief that women were somehow different, but we couldn't quite define our conviction, or even verbalize it without being accused of female chauvinism, "reverse" sexism, or wishful thinking based on a naive view of the innate goodness of women. So there was an immediate and predictable scramble by all kinds of social scientists to study female practitioners, and the new young women electing to join them.

There was certainly a large body of myths permeating society about the stereotypic woman doctor. You've heard most of them. Commonly known as "Ol' Horseface," she was portrayed with sensible shoes, floral housedresses, and a neatly braided, tightly netted occipital bun. There were myths about women who distracted the men in their classes from study by overt or covert seduction. There were myths about women who capriciously dropped out of school to have babies, after destroying career chances for more deserving males who'd been forced to make way for them just because they were smarter. There were myths about women who frittered the taxpayers' money away by behaving like "wimmen" in all aspects of their personal and professional lives. We especially disliked the one about how mean and nasty older women were to younger ones.

The main objective of the social research was to find out the facts about the professional and life choices of women physicians as compared with their predecessors. Women of my generation were put down for having gone into the traditional "three P's": psychiatry, pediatrics, and public health. Usually these putdowns came from the surgeons, gynecologists, and others in lucrative and prestigious specialties who had kept their residencies firmly closed to these women. Also denigrated were women who maintained families and home lives by working irregular hours, part time, or even not at all during periods of childbirth and young family raising. They were considered second-class citizens by the very men who'd never had to make a bed or order a six-pack of tomato juice by themselves. With the increase in numbers, would the new women in medicine be able to do some professional trailblazing? Or would they continue to follow the old patterns?

The best way for you to obtain more information about the present and past history of women in medicine is simply to ask the librarian of your nearest medical school to point you to the *Cumulative Index Medicus* and give you a quick lesson on how to use it. (Librarians are the best people to have as friends, by the way; they are invariably helpful and patient with students.) If you can, also read the studies done by Marilyn Heins and her colleagues in Detroit, who questioned large numbers of women physicians about how they managed their homes and families, along with their careers. The results should have meaning for you.

They found, for example, the following: Women physicians moved more often than men physicians, relocating their work more frequently, and interrupting their training as well. Although they had more training than men, fewer of them were "board certified," a status relating directly to income and prestige. More than twice as many women as men worked for somebody else. They held far fewer top-level administrative jobs, or jobs in government and medical education. (At the time of this writing, there is not a single full-time female dean of a medical school in the United States.) Fewer women than men belonged to professional organizations, and worked for them less often when they *did* join. Women were more self-effacing than men: It was impossible to get accurate figures about whether or not women worked as long or as hard as men, because men tended to include their "on call" hours, and women tended to overlook all their informal and volunteer assignments!

Most remarkable of Dr. Heins's findings involved women's perceptions of stress in their lives. In a recent article in the *American Journal of Public Health*, I summarized some of this material and did a wrap-up of my own:

> When asked about work overload, three times as
> many men as women felt that office pressures were

the reason, with women attributing pressure to home and child care rather than professional responsibilities. Three times as many men as women felt they should cut down on work at the office, while nearly 50 percent of the women felt they needed more help at home. Although 70 percent of the women physicians reported having domestic help at least one day a week, 76 percent said they do all the cooking, shopping, child care, and money management. Nearly 100 percent of women physicians have the responsibility for virtually all household tasks, whereas male physicians had none.

When questioned as to stress, 36 percent of the women and 15 percent of the men mentioned "conflict between work and outside life." Almost twice as many women as men (94 percent to 57 percent) perceived conflicts between career and traditional role relationships with members of the opposite sex. However, significantly fewer women (18 percent) than men (63 percent) expressed general feelings of stress about working too much. Lastly, more women than men felt they needed to modify themselves in some way.

Examining the implications of these data, we find ourselves confronting recurrent and contradictory themes.

On the one hand, we have an image of the average older woman physician today: She is the aggressive product of discriminatory admissions policies; qualified, productive, yet lower paid; has slower career advancement and recognition; and is clearly committed to home and family responsibilities deemed worthy of major professional sacrifice. She is underrepresented in all seats of power, less active in the public arena, depends on someone else

for her paycheck, and is politically uninvolved. She
tends to undervalue her own clout, blames herself
when caught in the crunch, and is still a servant to
her household. There is a good natured, self-effacing, plodding, salt-of-the-earth type image coming
across from these findings.

On the other hand, we have the new woman
physician. She is a composite of egalitarian principles, and her husband knows which end of the
diaper pin is up. A product of a role-liberating
society that made her career a matter of course
rather than another breakthrough, she can meet her
classmates twenty years hence without having to
ask them, "Did you ever get married? How old are
your kids?" Because all her energies will not have
been spent desperately scrounging flex-time residencies, day care, household help, self-regulated
working hours, a raise, an academic appointment,
tax advantages, and a piece of the power pie, she
may be given an opportunity for the first time since
women were admitted to medical colleges to show
what she can do as a physician—not just a "woman"
physician.

The question concerning us is "What is she going to do with it?"

The conclusion was that the future of women in medicine, and
their power to effect meaningful change in the way medicine is
practiced in the United States, depended upon the extent to
which they would be "co-opted" by their male colleagues, the
force of the overt establishment backlash in coming years, and the
flexibility and fortitude with which women would react to the two
issues.

If you are a woman contemplating medicine as a career, you
cannot afford to remain ignorant of the social and emotional

forces that will continually influence your acquisition and utilization of professional skills. You are walking into a hotbed of political and social foment, and it is your duty to be a part of it.

The classic mistake many dedicated women have made is to state that they do not consider themselves as women, only as doctors. This seems a public declaration of their devotion to science above all else, but it is actually a statement of denial, blindness, and pathetic illusions. Any woman who contemplates going into medicine without studying the recent literature about the experiences of women like herself ought to have her head examined. There is no point in reinventing the wheel, particularly when all the spokes are pointed at *her*! Furthermore, any woman who receives career counseling *exclusively* from men, and doesn't track down as many women as she can, will not be getting the comprehensive advice and counsel to which she is entitled. *Medicine is no profession for a woman who doesn't know exactly what she is getting into!*

The issue of whether or not women belong in medicine was settled well over a century ago, despite the near-eradication movement of the turn of the century. But only now are we beginning to find out how great a price women should have to pay for that undisputed right to belong. Let me explain what I mean.

In the old days, a woman could be a great physician simply by giving up everything else in life. If she was willing to travel anywhere, give up the demands of a family, spend her total life in service, she was accepted, honored, and given rich emotional rewards through service transactions many women found deeply fulfilling and rewarding. I knew many such marvelous old women during my training days. Yes, some of them *did* have horse faces! And they would have been amazed at the notion of wearing anything but a comfortable, easily washable dress, or laced-up Oxfords with square heels. But they were our pioneers, our "Phase I" of medicine, and each one should be treated as a national treasure.

In the fifties, along came a younger generation, however. Let's call them "Phase II." These women were not content to give up everything, especially things feminine, and insisted on having both career *and* family. They were the ones who were directly responsible for the development of the by now well-known "Superwoman" image. I described these women for *Medical Dimensions* in December 1977, in an article entitled "The Making of Superwoman."

For these women, I wrote:

> The mind had been developed like a steel trap, and the casing was packaged to enhance rather than conceal it. The woman physician of the fifties was expected to be a one-woman multipurpose service center. The assumption was that there were to be no renunciations in either her personal or professional life. From the moment she entered her training, the student would be able to handle everything well.
>
> The models held up to us were women who looked good, dressed smartly, maintained the interest of a husband, and were respected by their first-grade children, who proudly block-printed "doctor" in the space that said "mother's occupation." These women were expected to maintain their two worlds with verve and aplomb. Husbands were trained to pick up the kids with measles from the school nurse if mommy was in the OR, but otherwise were not be be overly burdened with domestic activity. PTAs were to expect contributions, not home-baked cakes, and to relieve these particular mommies of the obligation to man booths. At social events, women doctors were to enjoy passing incognito among the guests as "Mrs. so and so" . . . although it was understood that behind their backs, the whisper would pass: "She's a *doctor*, too!" If any

conflict leaked through publicly, it was considered bad form and a terrible example. Of course, there were lesbians, too—and no doubt they were very successful at that as well.

For our models, being a good engineer and administrator was as important as being a good diagnostician. It was cricket for a woman to impound female relatives and hired hands to support her in the professional style to which she was accustomed. A woman who did her own household scutwork, however enjoyable and relaxing, was deemed to be taking service from suffering patients, who could have made better use of her state-financed time. A woman had to be able to juggle budgets, office hours, broken appliances, kids' shopping jags, and the nocturnal labors of other women with the ease of a Moscow Circus performer rotating a family of six acrobats twenty feet above the seesaws.

The acid public test of a woman's capacity to combine both worlds came at delivery time, when a more-stoic-than-thou attitude pushed women into seeing who could work the longest before their pains made them run shrieking from the office. I distinctly remember two recently delivered residents in internal medicine one-upping on how dilated they were before they had to sign off the ward.

Superwoman dared not fail, for to do so was to give a black eye to all women physicians, who, like recently emigrated ethnic groups, were ultrasensitive to criticisms dealing with supposed collective traits considered unpleasant to the mainstream—in this case, male physicians. If at any point a woman lost her footing, her super-ego nagged: "What would the *men* say? We must be as good as, or better than, they are! We must ask for nothing they would not ask for! We must show them we can do it! We must be better women than they are men." This was invariably true in direct proportion to the vehemence with which she consciously denied it.

If a woman did *not* have home or family, and thus perpetuated the legend of her professional grandmothers, she was no less respected. She just went into another category. It was assumed, often erroneously, that a woman's single state was due to dedication, as opposed to other more immediate factors, such as unattractiveness, neurosis, bad luck, or even her unusual qualities and intelligence. A safe haven was provided for women such as these, so that personal bitterness should not diminish their professional effectiveness.

Although the goals and ideals of Phase II still permeate the thinking of most women in medicine (and other business and professional women, too), there are signs of movement into a "Phase III." This is a period in time in which a balance must be found between the aggressive career pursuits of late Phase II (i.e., increased solo, fee-for-service, private practice medicine in lucrative, hitherto closed specialties) and the growing awareness that "liberation" in career opportunities has not solved all the human problems. Compromise and reevaluation will have to become the hallmarks of Phase III.

Phase III is difficult to discuss because it takes us into unknown and controversial territory. It is an area in which it is almost impossible to be totally honest. We risk alienating and negatively mobilizing the male establishment with which women must coexist, antagonizing the feminists to whom we owe a debt that must be repaid, and shaking up our own innermost prejudices and defenses. Phase III is a tug of war between the compelling need to take advantage of all that has been offered to us, and the equally compelling need to stay ourselves and keep our lives under control.

Phase III is also hard to study. The only impression we have of it at the moment is accepted thought, which is a mixture of fact, dogma, impression, and easy packaging. All of these are inadequate to deal with the issues involved. After all, we are dealing with the vested interests of women who have predicated their lives on a philosophy of dual accomplishment at any cost, and will have trouble accepting any implication that sometimes even the best-oiled gears simply grind to a halt.

Some young women being counseled today about coming into the profession are still being clobbered with how difficult it is, in a tone reminiscent of Phase I. They are selectively advised to put their personal lives in cold storage and be prepared for a long, hard siege, advice rarely given in such bleakness to their male classmates. Others, primarily those who have had more opportunity to talk to practicing women physicians, are told that if they will but be supermanagers, they can have their cake and eat it, too. Books about "the woman manager" are pressed into their hands. In true Phase II style, they are urged to marry a "supportive" husband, experiment with role change and chore sharing, plan their families around their careers, get adequate household help, have money if at all possible, and order their lives with the infinite care of the Superwoman. In fact, there are by now a very large number of women physicians who have successfully managed to live dual lives, and it is now an accepted fact that medicine need not be a sentence of all work and no play.

But Phase III must soon deal with the fact that for *some* (please note, I said some) women, it is not enough to be a supermanager. As every reformed Type A personality can tell you, there comes a time when efficiency, organization, and minute-splitting simply isn't enough. Sooner or later, a woman will have to deal with the constant stress of living a dual life. She may have to consider a reduction in aspirations and accomplishments in both personal and professional spheres to bring her life into harmony, and to keep the stress consistent with her ability to cope.

The thought of any "cutbacks" in unlimited female role expansion is a heretical idea. It is this thought that many feminists see as the betrayal of their cause, and that men will seize upon to support their contention that women should stick to less demanding professions. Women who have fought for years for the right to develop Type A personalities, and bronchogenic carcinoma from smoking like men, will not wish any acknowledgment that some curtailment of upward striving and its concomitants may be right and necessary, and need not be signs of weakness or regression. Men who have insisted that women belong in the kitchen and not in the laboratory will see any suggestion that one person simply cannot be in both these places at the same time as confirmation that women should stick to just one—and you know *which* one!

Life for women physicians must have been simpler under Phase I, where there were virtually no options. There was no school nurse to call and say, "Mary Lou has the measles; please come and take her home," right in the middle of office hours, for there was no Mary Lou, and no husband to help share the load of chauffeuring a six-year-old little girl with fever and a rash.

Life became more complicated, and certainly more rewarding, under Phase II, when choices began to open up, even dumb ones like, "Who's going to go pick up Mary Lou?" Utilitarian solutions often worked.

But Phase III, with its dizzying freedom and embarrassment of alternatives, must surely cause the greatest personal stress. In Phase II we have settled that the *housekeeper*, of course, will pick up Mary Lou, but we will now revive some old questions for new answers. Who will deal with the anxiety? Should it have been a parent to go for Mary Lou in her hour of need, rather than a hired hand? And what happens when the housekeeper is off visiting her relatives in the Caribbean, or didn't show today, or gave notice that she is quitting at ten this morning because she got a better job elsewhere? Is it wise to become indebted to baby-sitting in-laws whose services were taken more for granted back in the unliberated fifties? Which parent gets stuck with these decisions?

You might enjoy reading some of the letters that were elicited in response to the Superwoman article. They certainly give some flavor of what life can be like for dual-role women in Phase III.

> From a psychiatrist in her mid-forties:
> . . . How well I remember those women who have served as my role models. I am referring in partic-ular to the pediatric and ob-gyn staff at school. They really did it all, and made it seem relatively simple. As I am living through a rather difficult time in my life (divorce), I was heartened to read your description of the less-than-perfect woman physician. I thought I had to be Superwoman. Now I know I have to be me. I am less than perfect, but much happier realizing it. . . .

> From a physician in California:
> . . . The Superwoman image has been a problem to me in recent years, when, after marrying and reproducing late, I found myself trying to fill all roles well and not quite making it. I look around at my approximate contemporaries to see how they are juggling all these chores. I haven't found any good answers. There are the Superwomen you described, running themselves ragged, working full time, entertaining at home, "raising" three kids, on call every other night, cranky and cantankerous master sergeants I don't want to copy. Those who have tried part-time work find many disappoint-ments: Uninteresting work may be all that's avail-able, fringe benefits are crummy, advancement is limited.
> I felt I was faced with a dilemma when my

salary was raised abruptly at the beginning of the affirmative-action move. I gathered I had been underpaid relative to the men in the department, but I didn't want to work their version of full time, which included Saturdays. Now I feel guilty accepting full-time pay and not working Saturdays, but if I work less than full time, out go the fringe benefits!

It seems difficult for women in medicine to get together in friendly fashion, having such guilt-laden versions of what they should be and what they are. Among my doctor supervisors, the least sympathetic to my desire to lead a reasonable life is a female superachiever, who seems to be saying, "If *I* can do it, why the hell can't you? I have three kids! I take call every other night! Do your share!"

Maybe this is why the American Medical Women's Association has limited appeal to younger people—too many generation and attitude gaps. I teach in a medical school, and tremble for the naiveté of the women who think that today's young men are all that enlightened, or that enlightenment itself will make a change in demands. Their husbands, if they marry, are likely to be the sixty-plus hour/week physicians (or other professionals), male versions of superachiever, and the household and kids will fall somewhere in the abyss between the two towering careers. I agree that things will never be quite even. Your lively article helps me to accept what I was coming to believe, that I cannot do it all and do it well, not at this point in my children's lives. . . .

From a physician in New Jersey:
. . . I, too, am a graduate of your medical school, and my experience was much the same as yours.

We, too, were raised that we could and should have equally successful home and professional lives. Would you believe we even had lectures on the subject? And these were comforting to many, too. We needed reassurance that though we were training to be doctors, being feminine, being mothers and wives were not mutually exclusive. Little did we realize the schizophrenic existence ahead. . . .

I am now one of those Superwomen that you alluded to. I have a husband, two children, and a practice, not in that order. At the moment, I am the sole breadwinner in the family. I am accepted most of the time and respected. My professional name and married name are the same. I am not threatened by the occasional patients who call me "Mrs.," that's a respectable title, too. But there are only twenty-four hours a day and there is absolutely no way I could be chairperson of anyone's department of medicine and be a mommy at the same time. So far, my kids don't resent me, but they're still very young. In fact, my daughter thinks all women in white are doctors and she wants to be one, too. It's my own guilt that pulls me home to make sure that I put my children to sleep at night. Doctor daddies don't do this.

Perhaps the new part-time training programs will ease things a bit, as will the growing awareness that there's nothing wrong with fathers pushing shopping carts, soothing tears, and changing diapers. Perhaps, too, there's a future for groups of women in practice together, on a part-time basis with complementary hours and times off. It sure beats twenty-four hours a day at home. God knows, I'd starve as a typist. But on the other hand, have you ever wished you could be bored for just one day? The idea intrigues me no end, but alas, I've no experience!

From a physician in the South:
. . . I am in my mid-thirties, a graduate of Harvard Medical School in full-time specialty practice. I have been divorced for a few years, after a five-year marriage, and am the mother of a young child. My ex-husband was a classmate who left me for another woman, one not quite so equal and therefore, I guess, less threatening, more gratifying. Meantime, working against me for remarriage or a relationship with another man is my age, my membership in an elite profession, and my status as a divorcée and mother of a young child. Where does one find those wonderful men who genuinely adore bright women?

From an intern in the Midwest:
. . . I am thirty-one, doing a rotating internship at the local city hospital, unmarried, and have felt and gone through just about everything you write about. I went to Michigan State University College of Human Medicine, a very supportive school with a high percentage of women students, women faculty, and a heavy emphasis on communication and relationships. It took a year or so for the men in our class to become accustomed to us, but they did, and became our staunch defenders. Still, most of them looked for nurses to love, and we women have remained on our own. . . . I'm going into surgery, and the surgeons are the last bastion of chauvinism and supremacy. . . . The other women I work with understand completely what you say.

The men, of course, will not. The angriest woman I know is a black intern—she feels totally isolated here. . . . I'm proud of the person I am, and work to be proud of the physician I am. I wouldn't change for anything, but, damn it, it gets so lonely sometimes. It hurts a lot to see my major male peer group go trotting off with the nurses. It also hurts to see some of the fine older physicians satisfied with the women to whom they are married. . . . The number of women in medicine is increasing again, and the effect of our presence will be very interesting sociologically. A couple of months ago a resident's wife said to him, "I hope I never lose you to one of those nurses at the hospital." At the time he was having an affair with a woman physician and is seriously considering divorce, a situation I am certain will become more common. I do not rejoice in the breakup of a family, but I sometimes feel pity for the women who are so comfortable being dependent. Thanks for expressing the collective pain and rage we have, as well as the pleasure and joy. . . .

From an American woman physician in Israel:
. . . Somewhere along the line I remember a study done by the Radcliffe Institute in the early sixties comparing the staying power of women in medicine with that of men. The results were quite contrary to the mythology about women dropping out. Indeed, as I recall, the average woman doctor gave significantly more years to medical practice than her male contemporary. I'm afraid I can't recall where these data were published. I just remember schlepping the paper around with me to all my internship interviews, waiting for the inevitable

moment when the interviewer would fix me with a beady stare and ask me, "How do we know you won't get married in the middle of your internship and go off to have babies?" or something equally infuriating. I would thereupon triumphantly produce the data showing that the male dropout rate from medicine was considerably higher than that for females and, furthermore, that men were much more likely to drop dead inconveniently at an early age, etc. It was wonderful ammunition, and no woman applicant to medical school or residency should be without it, even today, with affirmative action and all that. . . . I am reminded of the time a very gung-ho feminist reporter from the Pittsburgh *Press* came to interview me for an article about women in medicine (I was supposed to be role model of the week, no doubt), and found me vacuum-cleaning my apartment. She was scandalized, and I could not convince her that even role models have to do a little housecleaning now and then. . . .

Since the primary concern of many young women going into medicine is the feasibility of combining a career with a home and family, the first consideration is whether or not choosing medicine impedes a woman's chance of *finding* a husband. There is no easy answer to this question, since we obviously are in a period of great transition. In the past, statistics have shown that women in medicine tended to marry later than other women, and had fewer children and later; they also showed that fewer women married at all. A large percentage of my all-female class at medical school was still unmarried ten years after graduation. However, we do not know how much these figures depended upon chance, circumstance, or the personalities of the women involved.

Probably any woman who wishes to marry can do so, be she

doctor, lawyer, or Indian chief. However, Phase III's problems can influence her, even early in the game. Several years ago, I wrote some columns about the difficulties imposed on women who wanted to study medicine, but who also wanted to date like normal people—spontaneously, relaxedly, frequently, and purposefully. It was important to be frank about the problems I perceived, so I included a pretty heavy description of them. The articles provoked a lot of anxiety and controversy, because they evoked too much of Phase III.

I pointed out that at a time in life when many women were out there playing the field, going skiing in winter, beach-hopping in summer, the woman medical student and pre-medical student was up to her auricular orifices in textbooks, foul-smelling lab specimens, and library stacks. She rarely had time to date, and usually couldn't relax when she did. She had no time for long hot showers, browsing at cosmetic counters, hitting the sales on designer clothes, or keeping *au courant* with the latest disco beats. Young women were reminded that their relative inaccessibility and inflexibility in dating situations worked to their disadvantage, particularly in those areas where dating was a socially competitive phenomenon. Perhaps there was more than a grain of truth to the maternal wail, "Who'd want to marry a woman doctor?"

It also seemed necessary to acknowledge the fact that women were changing as they passed through the years of their education. They were becoming more sophisticated, more discriminating, more demanding in finding men who could be good companions intellectually and feel comfortable with a highly successful, extravagantly educated wife. As their need developed for men who could keep up with them, their less-pressured former classmates were picking them off, one by one, into holy wedlock. Although a number of women physicians were able to find fellow physicians and other professionals with whom they could live, others couldn't. Most male physicians did not seriously consider their female classmates as potential mates, preferring to date women with whom they felt they could let their hair down. It seemed frustrating and unsatisfactory, but very true, that women physicians were indeed not considered prime candidates for marriage by men who preferred women who would care for them, look up to them, and not compete in any sense for their time, loyalty, or affections.

The storm of letters in response to these observations confirmed impressions that a nerve had been hit. Part of the Superwoman mystique was that women physicians, if properly organized, could do anything. Who wanted to admit that establishing a love relationship with a marvelous man was something that simply could not be *willed* into existence? Who wanted to admit to the threatening idea that men simply could not be counted on to love accomplished, fearfully organized women? And how many women could admit to the fact that they, like their male colleagues, had grown accustomed to issuing orders and being unquestioningly obeyed, then had trouble giving it all up in a social relationship?

Although these problems were not insurmountable, and no woman had to be doomed to enforced loneliness, it seemed important to offer a realistic view of the competitive social marketplace for men who were in a position to take home anyone they wished in matrimony.

Following are some excerpts from this particular article.

> Despite the current marriages and the development of alternative arrangements, most women are married by the age of twenty-five and the probability of marrying for the first time goes steadily downward beyond that age. The suicide rate for unmarried women physicians of forty is shockingly high, higher than for physicians in general, already a high-risk group. Although much of the recent literature rightly deals with the problems of physician wives and mothers, we could use a little more discussion of the needs of women who have trouble

connecting with men who can make them happy.

Women physicians don't have to marry for the traditional reasons. They have no need of money, status, prestige, or the other things that attract women who cannot provide these for themselves. When a woman physician marries, her choice is infinitely less contaminated by extraneous factors. Who knows? Perhaps it is this rather than her prolonged education that keeps her single for so long. In any event, an otherwise laudable discriminatory sense can outfox her, if it is too critically exerted.

Remember, we are not discussing women who decide for good and valid reasons—or even for bad or neurotic ones—that they just don't want to get married. I speak to the woman who does want to marry, but feels she has all the time in the world, and other priorities at the moment. It chills my erythrocytes when I hear medical students say that they "don't want to get involved just now." If not now, when?

Women committed to an exclusionary ideal would do well to recognize that no one is allocating a portion of the best men for them, or keeping them in storage for release on demand.

Perhaps you would be interested in reading some more of the responses to the issues that had been raised?

From a woman physician in California:
. . . One of the aspects of being single while in training which I found difficult was the practice of signing up for further training so far ahead of time. And if your best career opportunity was in another city, it compounded the problem. It would be socially acceptable to cancel a residency commit-

ment because one just got *married* to someone who had to stay in another city, but it would be difficult to say that you are suddenly refusing to go to your residency in Albuquerque or wherever (as you promised over a year ago) because you just met an interesting man a few weeks ago and want to see how things turn out. The dilemma has faced a couple of my friends. Others have just stayed in one city, afraid to commit themselves far in advance. Of course, men have problems with commitments in advance, too, but their social position allows them to have more control over their social lives. . . .

From another woman physician in California:
. . . I'm thirty-one years old, married to a widower with three children, and have two of my own in addition. My specialty is anesthesiology. . . . I do hope in the future that some stroke of luck will make it possible for women and men, too, to become "whole" persons rather than the narrow academic-minded, typical medical student that our jealous profession has demanded in terms of our time and how it is to be spent. . . . In my mind, being a woman in medicine has been like having my cake and eating it, too. I wouldn't have wanted to marry a different kind of man regardless of my education and financial independence created by being a doctor. It would be lowering one's standards for the sake of conforming. But then women in medicine do march to a different drummer and therein lies the problem—it probably isn't our careers that interfere, just our attitude toward life in general.

From a male physician in Pennsylvania:
. . . Your article should be required reading for all

female medical students. . . . You refer to the problem of trying to "connect" with a suitable mate. The proverb, "It is better to give than receive," looks at the problem another way. It seems better to me to try to connect with someone I can make happy rather than someone who can make me happy. Both are important, of course, but the different emphasis makes me work harder in a relationship. . . .

From a woman physician in New Jersey:
. . . I am a woman surgeon, which perhaps makes me even more formidable, and I was single until the age of thirty-five. . . . Now as far as marrying a doctor, that's the last thing that I ever entertained in my mind. Statistics have shown that the highest incidence of divorce is in the doctor-to-doctor marriage, and that the clash of careers that occurs can be very devastating. This is not to say that it never works, because in many cases it does very successfully; I have many friends who are married to physicians and doing just fine. But it takes a lot of tolerance and understanding on both sides, and I think those of my friends, like myself, who are married to men other than physicians are much better off in the long run.

. . . My concern was not lack of males, it was a lack of males who I felt were of strong-enough character not to want to be continuously leaning on me. . . . I went through two engagements because of this. . . . How did I solve the problem? By diversity! By diversity, I mean one had to first get away from medicine, and move out into wider social circles where you can get a chance to meet the man who is going to meet your expectations.

> I thus eventually met a writer of national renown
> who filled the bill. . . . What I'm trying to say is
> that you have to get away from medicine. It's fine
> to be dedicated to medicine, but I feel that to be
> a whole, well-rounded person, you need interests
> outside of it. I never had time to be lonely because
> I was too busy doing things. . . .

Perhaps this discussion of the social lives of women in medicine hasn't concerned you particularly. That's OK. I only wanted to stress that Phase III means that stereotyped methods of dealing with complex human issues just won't do. Be aware!

A great deal can be learned from the letters quoted here. All the writers had personally grappled with the problems of reconciling a heavy schedule and emotional commitment to the equally demanding necessity of having a firm emotional life and people to love. No two had solved their problems in the same way. Some had done better than others! But none had escaped the need to find a road that took them two places at once.

It seemed to me that the best way to illustrate the unknowns and hazards of Phase III would be to offer a "case example" of one woman who'd been plunged into it. And then, by sheer coincidence, a call from a young woman physician friend resulted in a long, two-hour bull session. As I listened to her talk, and tried to cut through some complicated details to get to her problem, I realized that she was enduring conflicts that offered a crystal paradigm of the problems facing women in training today.

Here's her story. Rachel is about twenty-nine and presently a second-year resident in internal medicine at a major medical center in a metropolitan area. I met her seven years ago, as she was completing several years of graduate school in a medically related field. We became friends when I moved into the apartment next door to hers, and she baked me a cake. I was happy to hear that she was considering medicine as a career, and gave her a big, fat push, because she was smart, attractive, well motivated, warm-hearted, and a simply delightful person. She went through an anxious year of rejections because she was late in applying, but tried again successfully the following year.

During her four years in school, I was able to watch her career from a proximity granted to few but parents and spouses. Each night she'd come home and share her experiences with her husband, with me, and the rest of her friendly neighbors, some of whom were doctors themselves. Luckier than many, she received much support and expert advice. Her husband genuinely applauded her aspirations and wanted only her happiness. Her friends knew how to orient her, saving much scutwork and time-wasting. Nothing could spare her the trauma of exams and grades and the ubiquitous fear of failure, but she graduated with a respectable average, a residency at a good hospital not far from the suburban home she'd recently purchased—and a baby.

A doctor in training *never* finds the right moment to have a baby, but insofar as these things can be planned, this baby came at the perfect time. My friend saved up all her vacation time for the six-week period before and after her delivery, in September of her senior year. She arranged to take her easiest electives during the months immediately before and after that vacation period. In all, she had close to six months of free or undemanding time.

She had many other things in her favor, too. Her husband was a successful businessman, which meant that she had no insurmountable money problems. Money can't buy happiness, but it can buy help, time, and support. She was able to hire a competent, live-in child-care person, whose major responsibility was the baby, not the house. (She obtained cleaning help as needed.)

As if born under a happy star, my friend had a mother-in-law who lived nearby and loved her as dearly as a daughter. Many were the days when this woman would "just drop by" with a freezerful of homemade goodies, thereby taking care of cooking needs for a full week. And once I remember she brought back an armload of clothes on approval from one of the city's finer shops, so that "the doctor" could make a decision without having to sacrifice a minute of precious study time! May we all have such mothers-in-law.

It was safe to say that during her four years as a medical student, my friend's experiences with sexism, prejudice, and bias against women were minimal. Her school had a fairly liberal reputation, professors nowadays know enough not to project cheesecake anatomy slides, and her savvy group of friends could maintain a healthy, moderately antiestablishmentarian attitude that protected them from too much trauma. And so it was with high hopes that she began her career as a doctor.

She knew it would not be easy. An intern is suddenly plunged into those three or four postgraduate years without much sense of his or her capacity to perform as a *real* doctor. Fatigue sets in. The skills that must be acquired are great. But she was prepared to give it her all, knowing that her household was functioning smoothly, her child was left with a trained individual, her support system was strong, and her husband was prepared to be the most attentive and loving parent a kid could possibly have.

My friend started the dizzying round of being up all night, night after night, being plunged into uncertainty, consumed with feelings of ineptitude, and calling home at crazy moments just to hear her ten-month-old cry "mama" into the phone, and hear her husband say, "All's well here, kid, no sweat!"

During that first postgraduate year, we saw each other far less frequently, for although we now lived near each other again, in our own homes, it wasn't like the old days when our front doors were only inches apart. Also, we were both busy, a poor backdrop for maintaining intimacy. Instead we talked on the phone, her weary voice describing her adjustment. These calls were accompanied by a lot of background noise and were frequently cut off by a page, or a quick and unexplained, "Hey, can I call you back?" There was no doubt that my friend was soon deep in the throes of the old, intern, when-am-I-going-to-feel-like-a-human-again? blues.

Things *did* seem to be going well at home, thanks to her Superwoman planning. She was good-natured and not jealous when people remarked that her husband was as good as a mommy! She humorously reported that people were teasing her by asking if the kid recognized her when she came home. And it was obvious that the little girl, who was as darling as both of her parents, looked like both of them, loved both of them, and showed how nicely she was being nurtured by being an engaging, bright, and seemingly totally normal little person.

At the beginning of her second postgraduate year (the first year of her residency), she began thinking about choosing a specialty. Exhausted from her first year, it was understandable that her decision would be based in no small part upon how much time and energy the field would take, how compatible it would be with raising a family, and how long it would keep her in training before she could get out on her own. All residents go through something like this, particularly in internal medicine, where a subspecialty choice can be as serious as earlier decisions.

When she called a few nights ago, her voice all stressed out, I'd no idea that her conflict over this decision would be anything more than the usual. I was deep in the middle of writing Chapter Seven, but she needed a sounding board, and what are friends for? I put up a pot of tea, made some feeble efforts to straighten out the mess in the den, and waited for the doorbell.

She looked awful. Her eyes were absolutely glazed over. What should have been a simple career decision seemed to be invested with such tremendous emotional struggle it was obvious that she had more than one "hidden agenda" cluttering her mind. I listened as she poured out her conflicting options. Should she finish out her three years of internal medicine training and just be a generalist? She would always have the option of returning at some point in the future for subspecialty training. But, of course, it's always harder to come back, so wouldn't she be better off getting it over with now? But what should it be? And she was so tired! Should she just try to stall for time and decide later? But everyone else was deciding now, and if she procrastinated, she'd lose out on a residency that was highly competitive. And nothing seemed to interest her. Well, no, that wasn't true, *everything* interested her, but not enough to *specialize* in. But she had to choose *some*thing!

"I've changed my mind about dermatology and rheumatology," she said, alluding to two former enthusiasms. I noticed that she was twisting her fingers nervously around the ends of her hair. "I'm getting serious about anesthesia." I tried very hard not to change the expression on my face. The idea of a born internist sitting and passing gas all day was kind of hard to take with a straight face. "Please don't laugh," she begged, as if reading my thoughts. "Everyone is laughing at me about it. But it's really just right for me. I talked to some of the women in it, and they all say they get to go home at five every night, and they don't have to take any work home with them when they leave!" Her voice sounded full of anguished longing and, suddenly, a lot of her anguish became clear. Wow! Who would have thought it?

As if she felt that she had to convince herself as well as me, she went on to sing the praises of putting people to sleep, stressing how much intellectual work there really *could* be if she would just put her mind to it. (Quite unfairly, many people think of internists as the "brains" of medicine, and the anesthesiologists as those who want a relatively quiet existence.) Frankly, it was hard to recognize this confused apologist as the determined, obstacle-jumper I had known for so many years. She had changed. Only obliquely and very delicately could she talk about her desire to be at home more with her family, for it made her feel very guilty. It was hard for her to see that much of the anxiety to defend her latest career choice came from her unwillingness to accept her need for more of a personal life. She sounded like a woman who was being motivated into a career track by reasons that she sensed weren't valid, but were so compelling she had to give in. She also seemed to be reacting to a fear of criticism from her peers.

Well, one thing was certain. I respect deeply a woman's desire just to kill time with her child (useless, purposeless, unplanned, relaxed time), and *I* certainly wasn't going to criticize her for her blossoming feelings.

On the contrary, it was now *my* turn to feel guilty. For years I had been so happy to see good women go into medicine, I had downplayed the problems and radiated only unflagging enthusiasm. I had never wanted to frighten them off with lurid details of the hardships, nor had I wanted to impose my own doubts about what they were undertaking. I had heard that there were women who were hard on their younger sisters, perhaps from jealousy or some other morbid need to keep them down, and there seemed no more unpleasant way to behave. I also was not comfortable with discouraging people, or sharing my doubts with them, because I knew that we are all creatures with differing strengths and weaknesses, which meant differing capacities to handle stress. What one woman can handle well, another woman may find intolerable. It is unfair for the latter to try to dissuade the former.

But now I wondered if I were not partly responsible for what had happened to my friend. By my silence, had I been complicit in leading her down a difficult path? I asked myself, "If she had discussed possible pregnancy with me while in medical school, what would I have said? Would I have confessed that I did not see how I, personally, could ever have the strength to leave my own baby, day after day, no matter how much I loved my work? Would I have suggested that she hold off until she had completed her training, so that she could have a better chance of gaining control of her life? Or would I have stifled all my personal feelings and offered her only the happiness of a friend at her good fortune?" I realized that I would probably have taken the last road. And I felt guilty about it.

The questions were all hypothetical, of course. My friend had managed the timing of her pregnancy according to her own needs, which is perfectly appropriate, and she probably would have filed my opinion exactly where it belonged. Well, all of these thoughts flashed through my head as she went on trying to convince me that she was not crazy for suddenly wanting to make people unconscious. I jerked myself back to reality to try to deal with the problem she was presenting. *Should* she study anesthesia?

Who was I to offer an opinion? I hadn't been in an operating room in twenty years! It probably could be as good a specialty as any. But it was necessary to point out that if she was looking for a nine-to-five position, she certainly didn't have to take a residency in the big A to get it. There were many options in internal medicine that she had not explored at all, options such as working in a college student-health service, an industrial employee-health program, the insurance industry, any one of a number of group health or large partnership plans, or even the prison health system. (I also made a mental note to find out why she had not considered these obvious alternatives.)

Besides, she'd had very little practical experience with anesthesia, and there was no guarantee that she'd like it. Wasn't she going out on a limb to ensure a reasonable life for herself? What good would it do her to have decent hours if she did not enjoy the way they were being spent? She was making a career choice from a position of weakness, under conditions of extreme exhaustion. No good could come of it. Her best bet seemed to be to finish out her residency as originally planned, take a very long vacation, become a free agent again, and then make a decision about a job or further training when her spirit and enthusiasm had returned. It was just awful to see a woman who had gone through life with a bang end up with a twisted hank of hair, a muted whimper, and a canister of nitrous oxide to keep her company.

Once she agreed not to rush into anything, we could talk more about options. It was necessary because part of her depression and sense of being boxed in came from a feeling that she'd have to abandon her specialty, and a freely chosen subspecialty, to have flexibility of life-style. Where had she gotten that idea? It seemed important to find out. So I asked her to talk more about why she felt so hog-tied by the profession to which she had dedicated so much of herself.

Internal medicine was so vast, so huge, she said, how could one function and live with one's conscience without reading all the journals each night? And how could she read the journals if she wanted to spend her spare moments with her husband and little girl? So didn't that mean that if she stuck with this career, the more she gave her family, the less she'd give her patients? She couldn't bear that. In a conspiratorial tone of voice, implying that no one else must know, she confessed, "I haven't touched a journal in three months!" From this it naturally followed that she now wanted a specialty that was fairly circumscribed, so that she could master and stay on top of it without feeling overwhelmed and underprepared every day!

As she continued to talk, it became clear that she was dissatisfied with the way in which her training was being inflicted upon her. "I've come to hate internal medicine," she said bitterly. "I hate them for what they have done to me, to patients, and to themselves." I didn't have to ask who she meant by "they," or what it was they had done. I knew. She was reacting to the chauvinism, smashed ideals, and parochialism of the medical center. She was overwhelmed with the pressures, the demands to be perfect, the standards that seemed superhuman. A woman who should have been a very competent diagnostician and patient caretaker was being pushed off into a fairly "nonpatient-relating" specialty by the insensitivity and driving goals of her mentors. She seemed to be unaware that she was punishing herself by rejecting their specialty simply because she couldn't punish *them*. She was throwing her training out with the bathwater.

(It happens. In fact, it reminded me that I had once loved obstetrics, but had been so turned off by the horrendous behavior and attitudes of my teachers in medical school that I couldn't wait to get out of the delivery room permanently.)

Further discussion revealed that her mentors at the hospital were putting her under great pressure to specialize and telling her that if she did not, she would not rise to the top of her profession or command the kind of position that would avoid a professional dead end. She was being spurred to a pursuit of excellence that seemed to be out of all proportion to what a human being could be expected to acquire without going bananas. No wonder she felt utterly guilty playing with her baby when she thought she should have been reading the journals!

"Look," I said, "you were good enough to graduate from medical school when they could have flunked you out! You got a good residency and have functioned well for a year and a half! How big a butcher could you possibly be? Don't you know that you know as much or more than any young physician in your position? Don't you trust your own integrity to refer patients you cannot handle to another physician with more expertise in the problem? Do you really rank yourself with other doctors whose pride is so great they can't ask for help? And did it never occur to you that you could limit your practice to the kinds of patients with whom you feel most comfortable, that you do not have to be all things to all people?" It was hard to believe we still had to keep going through these basics.

All she needed was to have a satisfying career. And all this meant was taking care of sick people, having faith in her ability to care for them, and ensuring that she have reasonable time to spend with her family. She didn't have to become a superspecialist, a hospital chief, a power broker in the medical establishment, an academician, researcher, or scholar. She could have the quality practice she demanded without all of the above. There was a time when all she had wanted was to be a doctor. What had happened to her? Who had been working on her?

In part we can blame the "male" medical establishment, whose striving for performance (it is not always excellence) at times crosses the border of emotional disturbance. In part we can blame the influence of the women's movement, which has often pressured women beyond their own endurance, and often beyond that of the men with whom they work. And in part we can blame our own inner weaknesses, which make us prey to such self-punishing behavior. One woman was sitting in my den, with her feet up on the old blue end table, but every woman in medicine had a stake in our conversation.

I hope you are getting a feeling for the complexities of the issues, although I have discussed only a few of them here. In fact, I may not have addressed the most important ones! Who do you think was the real enemy? Who are the real villains, if there were indeed any at all? What was the real problem? We would have been wrong, don't you think, to approach this woman's dilemma by considering her just another mother who wanted to be with her baby? Wouldn't we also have been shortsighted to consider her a burned-out woman who was simply tiring of the prolonged strain? Nor would it have been enough to call her an idealist who'd been hurt and wanted only to retreat to the safe haven she called home. She was all of those things and more. She was a woman physician, deep in the throes of Phase III.

Lest you feel that I am painting some dire picture of a nervous wreck, let me assure you that this isn't so. I know my friend too well to believe that she is suffering anything more serious than a severe but temporary case of the wear-outs. Her professional aspirations may be momentarily dampened, but they are not irretrievably damaged by events. Many women go through similar experiences (and men, too). In many ways, she is lucky because she *does* feel conflicted and depressed. She can get her feelings out in the open, talk about them, and then find a way to resolve them. Some others are less fortunate, more limited in their emotional expression.

I know that my friend will have a very satisfying career, after all. She will probably finish out her residency, wisely playacting an enthusiasm she may not always feel to keep her supervisors off her back. She'll find the kind of position that will enable her to fulfill her resolution, "It won't be like this with the next child!" But I think her story is valuable for women toward whom she will someday feel as "big sisterly" as I feel toward her. (It's also valuable for men who will sacrifice everything in their climb to the top of medicine.)

Remember that many women will not share her experience at all. Many women in medicine don't marry until they are through with their training. (Since many women who want a career are now postponing marriage, they are no longer very different from other women!) Women who marry and have their children later in life have more autonomy in the management of their affairs.

Other women may not marry at all. Some women not only treat the early acquisition of a husband with contempt, but also extend their disdain to having children at all, which clearly simplifies their lives. Some women marry physicians with whom they can share an unusually fulfilling life. And more and more gay women are acknowledging their position even as they study medicine. The one thing these women have in common is that they are women in what is still a man's profession, and probably always will be. They would be wise to deal with this simple fact from the beginning of their career plans.

Many physicians who read this chapter may say, "Why did she have to go and spend so much time on one woman's problem? Why is she scaring women away just at the moment she says she wants more of them? With her for friends, who needs enemies?" I take that risk, because I believe honesty is the best tool to accomplish my purpose. I have found that younger people in this country are so starved for honesty, it's just about the only thing they prefer to the easy answer. Medicine offers no easy answers, but then whoever said that easy was rewarding? Now that I have done my best to scare you off, I hope you'll accept the challenge anyway. No matter what your race, religion, creed, ethnicity, personality, or taste in designer jeans, medicine needs good women. The more of us there are, and the better we care for ourselves, the greater the impact we can make on the health of the country.

11.
If
You Aren't
Mainstream . . .

I am writing this chapter because it needs to be written and not because I have the expertise to do it as well as it should be done. I also write it knowing that those who need it most will have least access to it. Perhaps those into whose hands it does fall will help in getting the message across to those who should hear what it has to say. It is addressed to all the minorities who feel that medicine belongs to the other world of which they cannot be a part. This includes not only blacks and ethnic minorities, but gays and the handicapped as well. Their needs are not similar, but their sense of the impediments that lie in their way unites them.

Medicine needs them all. For too long it has been the private preserve of those who from childhood could anticipate success and achievement. Our ability to serve people has been hampered by the insularity and impatience of people who have never suffered a hardship that is not of their own making. So it is my hope that this chapter will be of assistance to a wide variety of people whose presence in our profession would decidedly enhance its effectiveness. It is important for such people to know that their participation is not only tolerated from a sense of social justice, but actively welcomed for the very attributes that have been unapprcciatcd for so long. Let's start with young members of the black and ethnic communities.

The black middle class, and ethnics of the second and third generation who have "made it" by mainstream standards, will relate to this chapter as if they were part of that group. But they are not the population to whom I am speaking. If you are black, Hispanic, Chicano, native American, or Oriental; if you have known poverty; if you are bilingual; if you are intelligent and have a desire to make something of your life, you should be thinking seriously about medicine. I can well imagine that such a goal may seem out of the question for you. It takes money that you don't have, time that you can't afford, self-confidence that you still haven't developed, support from many people who may think you are overly ambitious, and luck that no one ever promised you. After all, look at all those rich white kids who didn't make it either.

If you are a woman or a younger son, you may well be under great pressure to stay home and cook, or go to work immediately to help support the family—perhaps even a more "chosen" relative who wants to study medicine himself. If you share the perception that you are indeed needed, you will have to add to your other worries some feelings of guilt over your familial abandonment.

Think about it anyway. Medicine offers you the same advantages it offers the American majority, and you are as much entitled to your piece of the pie as they are. It also offers you special satisfactions if you choose to work in the areas that need you most, the inner cities and rural, underserved communities. Of course, it offers you the same *dis*advantages, only more of them, and in more infinite variety!

My interest in the problem of recruitment of minority students into medicine was sparked when I joined the faculty of the residency program in social medicine of Montefiore Hospital in New York City. This was a very innovative graduate training program for young doctors who planned to work in the inner city out of

social principle. Many of them were Latino and black, and an unusually high percentage were minority women as well. (Do you remember that famous quote from Shirley Chisholm? She said that
she was a woman and she was black, and being a woman was
harder!) Our residents knew better than anyone else the need for
more docs like themselves.

One of our residents felt strongly that young blacks like himself
were systematically steered away from medicine, even as their
white counterparts were being indoctrinated, encouraged, and educated about the profession. He devised a rather ambitious program for educating junior-high-school students in inner-city areas,
planning to attend high-school assemblies and do some fancy talking. He also wanted to distribute some questionnaires to determine the level of understanding in tenth graders, so that he'd
know how to proceed. Because of the pressure of his own studies,
the common nemesis with generous schemes like this one, he was
not able to fulfill his ambitions. I have always wondered what he
might have been able to accomplish. Perhaps *you* could give it a
try!

The main reason that black and other minority students don't
think of medicine as a profession is simply that it is still a way of
life that belongs primarily to elite, white, ambitious, educated,
monied males. So what? Barriers have been falling left and right
in this country for years. You can hear the sounds of toppling
privilege all over the place, if you listen with an open ear. So why
not in medicine, too? You'll have to pick your way over some rubble, of course, and a weak structure or two may threaten to come
down on your head, but you can do a little ducking and make it
through to the other end.

When you do get there, you will find patients who will relate to
you as they do to no one else. They will be patients who can
speak to you without being misunderstood. They will be patients
who can tell you honestly what home remedies they have been
using, knowing that you will accept and not make fun of them, or
talk down to them. They will be patients whose needs you under-

stand like no other physician who has not shared or witnessed their hardships. You will be familiar with their beliefs, value systems, superstitions, customs, and ceremonies, and you will be able to use them to enhance the healing process for patients who are afraid and mistrustful of our cold, scientific, western medicine. Because by then you will recognize the value of both folk and scientific healing, you will be able to take what is good from each and use them both wisely.

One of our residents, an American-born Chinese, went down to Chinatown to work in a free clinic. There he undertook a study of Chinese medicine, which occupied and fascinated him as totally as his orthodox medical training! Before he had finished, he had had to sit down and learn the language of his ancestors. But now he is more useful than ten doctors, because he can experience the confidence of his patients, something a Caucasian physician might never win. Our Puerto Rican physicians also had an edge with their patients that made their colleagues quite envious. One of them spent a summer in medical school working with migrant workers in Michigan, establishing the first real health-care clinic they had ever known. Physicians like this, who are willing to teach the rest of us their customs and ceremonies, make us more effective in our work.

It is important for Caucasian patients to have the opportunity to consult minority physicians. It is not always easy for minority physicians to attend these people, for some will present all their biases and prejudices along with their varicose veins. Speaking as a woman physician who vividly remembers being thrown out of many a misogynist's sickroom, I can assure you that skilled care will win over a hate-filled bigot quite nicely. There isn't too much difference between the mentality that believes that a woman's place is in the kitchen and the mentality that believes that a black's place is scrubbing her floor. Treating such people is both a humanitarian and political necessity.

These are the problems of practice, however, and not as important as the problems of acquiring the education to deal with them.

Let's talk about some of the educational problems you'll have to deal with. The first thing that comes to mind is racism, pure and simple.

Racism. Medicine has its share. If it were the only racist profession, I'd say, "Why subject yourself?", but since it is really no worse than certain unions or other professions, why not go for broke? The racism of gentlemen is just as rotten as the racism of blue-collar workers, but it can be understood, handled, manipulated, ignored, even dismantled. Of course, racism in medicine is subtle. It can be cloaked in paternalism, layered over with intellectual horse feathers, excused in the name of academic purity, denied because it is so unacceptable to the people who exhibit it, and more hurtful because it comes from people you think should know better. But it's racism, impure and complex, and we are finding out a lot about what causes it, how it can be attacked, and what role it can or cannot play in breaking you. Racism should be nothing new to you. You've been handling it all your life and are not a complete babe in the woods. It's no different or worse at this level. My mother's favorite expression comes to mind, "Forewarned is forearmed."

It is not appropriate for me to give you lessons on handling racism. Still, although you will find no glib advice here about handling educators' negative feelings toward blacks and minorities, I can offer you whatever observations I have noted that may help.

The first item is dealing with your own racism. Believe me, if it weren't there, you could exhibit yourself as some kind of saint or something. Every time you hate someone from the mainstream because of his color or his position rather than his or her personal attributes, you're entering that world you will have to deal with when it spins around against you. Understanding and having the courage to face your irrational hatreds helps you understand others who put you down.

One technique that helps is simply recognizing that what binds people together is really much stronger than what separates them. This is even more true when ugly things bind them, like the lust for power, the desire for money and material attributes at all costs, and the need to get ahead no matter what the price. People are people. They use whatever they have. If *you* had the advantage, you might be just as rotten, and if *they* were in your shoes, they might just show even more sterling character than you possess. So try to think of even the most offensive individuals as being some image or mirror image of yourself, and you'll gain some sense of perspective.

Another technique that often helps is simply to get yourself outside of a painful situation and try to observe it the same way a journalist or social critic would. If you can become a social scientist, a recorder/reporter, an interpreter of events even as you are participating in them, a part of you will be forced to be objective about what is happening. It can be helpful.

Still another suggestion is for you to try to make your peace with the "Puritan ethic." Some people call it the "Protestant ethic." By whatever name you call it, it still refers to the old belief by the majority in this country that hard work pays off, that virtues are their own reward, and that good things happen to people who are willing to work, sacrifice, and have faith in their future.

Despite much cynicism, many believe in the Puritan ethic as a guiding force in becoming something that you want to be, no matter *who* you are, what your background, or what you want to be. Hard work, optimism, enlightened self-interest, staying as honest as you can in a rotten world, all these things give people a feeling of self-worth, accomplishment, and inner peace. This, in turn, helps them to handle what has to be faced in this world of ours. So don't throw it away too soon. It may not get you where you want to be, but you can't do much without it, if only because these are the values of the majority culture you wish to conquer.

Get guidance early. If you meet up with a racist, lethargic guidance counselor, run the other way. Many young people have been blindfolded and pushed in the wrong direction by school advisers who just didn't know how to pin the tail on their donkey. Look for a real mentor, someone you can trust, someone knowledgeable, preferably someone of your own color, background, temperament, and attitudes.

You will learn more techniques for handling the racism that permeates the entire medical-education process if you make it your business to find yourself such a mentor, as well as a group of people with similar aspirations who will provide support for one another. You don't know any black (or ethnic) doctors? Find them!

Call the National Medical Association, an organization of black physicians that's been around for forty years or more. Call your county medical society and ask them for a list of the black (or ethnic) doctors in your town. If you want to be more selective, call the office of the director of medicine at your closest university medical center or good "teaching" hospital (the one that has the best reputation and gets patients from all over). Talk to the director's secretary and ask for the name and phone number of the nicest, most responsive black (or ethnic) physician in the department, and state frankly why you are asking. Then get your body down to that doc's office and ask for whatever help you can get. Get books to read, names of people to meet. Find students from your neighborhood who'll let you spend a weekend while you get your nose rubbed in it. Talk about all the reality problems we'll be discussing in the next few pages. And make your move.

If you have the slightest interest in being a doctor, don't knock yourself out of the running without having made at least that one move of making a contact, and getting some practical help you just can't get from me. All I'm good for is telling you that it's possible, and it's hard.

I've talked about one of the problems racism. Let's talk about some more.

Lack of confidence. If you have read the preceding chapters, and not skipped immediately to this one, you will know by now that self-confidence is as rare among pre-medical and medical students as it is in a marine boot camp. Why should you be any different? Self-confidence comes with time and accomplishment, and you need only a small amount to get started.

I am recalling an incident recounted in an article entitled "The Vulnerability of the Medical Student." A black medical student was called upon to examine a young black girl. Unaccountably losing his cool and stammering all over the place, he even succeeded in introducing himself incorrectly! When asked about his gaffe after the incident, he said that he might have handled it differently had she been white. *"That girl knew who I was,"* he said. *"I felt as if I should be running the elevator, not trying to be a doctor!"*

It may take years for people to get over the destructive attitudes to which they have been subjected all their lives, but they have to make a start sooner or later. The past will always come back to haunt, but like many other painful things, it can be turned to good purpose. For example, consider the problems of a black woman resident who was enrolled in our program. We had scheduled a visit to the local office of the Human Services Administration (still known locally as "welfare") to try to give the group an understanding of the dehumanizing process to which their patients were subjected when they tried to obtain enough money to live. She became very agitated and flatly refused to go. *"I've seen enough welfare offices,"* she said firmly. *"How do you think I made it through the first sixteen years of my life?"* As the group stood in the hall, feeling terrible for her and even worse for themselves, she told us about her experiences with food stamps, dented tin cans, evicting landlords, etc. Everyone was the better for her candor, and she became a critical counterguide at the center to which she finally consented to go. This young woman had many adjustment problems in the hospital. She saw people who should have been seen as her colleagues as hated enemies and oppressors, in part because she could not break her old thought patterns and in part because their insensitive demands on her to "become white" helped to reinforce them.

For many students, the culture clash, which can be quite severe, is a major assault upon their integrity and self-confidence. Learning to make it in a foreign world is a stress no one should have to endure while undergoing the medical student "becoming" process, but it is there, and it has to be handled. If you believe you can do it, you have a valuable weapon—yourself. If you can learn to walk in both worlds; if you can keep what is good of your old world, and not let it conflict unnecessarily with the new, you will be doubly rich. You will also be twice as valuable to your patients, patients who come from both worlds. And if you can conquer your "survivor guilt," you can be a great help to the friends and relatives you left behind.

Money. Money is a problem for everyone. Going to college, and then medical school, is becoming more and more like getting a catastrophic illness: *No one* can afford it. The middle class may be hurting for the first time, but you always had it rough. What're a few big zero's, more or less? The average indebted medical student graduates with an educational debt of eighteen thousand dollars. For you, it may be even more. Don't worry about it. Just start hustling to find the bucks. Contact the National Health Service Corps branch office closest to you and go in for a talk. See if your state offers a free education if you will agree to serve local communities for a certain period of time after graduation. Get your librarians and guidance counselors at school to start digging up scholarship information for you. Start early. The poorer you are, the greater an edge you may have. Don't let big money stop you.

Many people who are able to find *big* money discover themselves in trouble over *little* money. I mean spending money—money earned from moonlighting at extra jobs, money borrowed to make ends meet after all the larger expenses are accounted for. Working and going to school can be rough, but it need not be a total wipeout. Get some guidance locally on this, too. Try not to lose medical school just because of money.

Feeling obligated. The United Negro College Fund once issued a very moving appeal for funds that showed an old grandmother scrubbing her heart out on office floors all night, so that her next generation could go to medical school. It should have been good for a lot of contributions, for it was real and very true. One could almost feel those arthritic knees creaking in the lonely chill of the abandoned corridors.

The other side of the coin, however, is that the recipients of this blood money are forced to bear an intolerable burden of gratitude and obligation. When beloved relatives, particularly those who are in no position to be suffering and sacrificing, are doing just that to ensure your chances for a better future, you have to be pretty insensitive not to have some real conflicts about subjecting them to it. I never said becoming a doctor was easy.

However, you should not lose sight of the fact that you bring a joy that money cannot buy to the hearts of those who sacrifice for you when you accomplish and succeed, and you do indeed represent an investment for the future. Each minority success is a success for an entire class of people, and therefore your pain and pleasure is not yours alone. Perhaps your conscience will be eased to know that for every doctor who succeeds, there are *many* who have worked to make the dream come true. It is not fashionable for people to sacrifice for others in today's world, but those who do it with a loving and uncalculating heart are still rewarded in a special way.

Feeling obligated is not related only to money borrowed or sacrifices made by loved ones. There is a special form of obligation that comes to those who are "representing" their race, their class, their sex, their families, or even their neighborhoods. ("He's the first kid from Pott's Corner ever to go to medical school!") The pressure to make good, to fulfill the expectations of others, to pave the way for younger people, to justify the favors performed, can be a real monkey on any student's back, but particularly a minority student's. It is important to learn to separate obligations, see them realistically, fulfill them according to your capabilities, and then dump them overboard when appropriate.

Burn out. Frequently, minority students who enter medicine with a strong desire to help their own people burn out in a special way. Having struggled and sacrificed for so long, they develop a particularly strong sense of entitlement, and want material rewards for their labors. These rewards do not come from returning to ghetto neighborhoods, where one is paid by Medicaid, Medicare, and gratitude. They do come from more comfortable practices, where people can forget where they came from for a while, or at least relegate it to a past they would prefer to remember than continue to experience.

Our residency program, which hoped to attract the best of the minority students, found them preferring the more prestigious centers of postgraduate education, the "big-name" hospitals. Our experience was similar to that of nearby schools of medicine, who found that minority students preferred going to Harvard and Yale. It is hard to blame them. In fact, minority students do have to protect themselves against being groomed to work only in ghetto areas. They have as much right to work where they please as others. Some settle for a compromise in which they divide their time between those patients who pay well and those to whom they feel a social obligation. Few escape the necessity of making some painful decisions. It is well known that doctors do not stay long in poverty areas, no matter what their color, unless they are extraordinarily dedicated.

All I can say to reinforce your finer instincts is to assure you that you bring to minority patients a wealth of background, empathy, and "street smarts" that few other physicians can ever really bring. That is an asset that should not be surrendered lightly.

Performing academically. Many minority young people are afraid that they just don't have what it takes to do the work. It is true statistically that you may have a poor educational background, and that there are too few supplementary programs to help you catch up. It is understandable that you may feel that everything is stacked against you, or that even if you do work hard to make it on your own, people will think that you got in just because of favoritism and quota systems. What do you care what people think? Your job is not to solve personally every civil and human rights issue confronting this country today. Your job isn't even to justify your own position and credentials. Your job simply is to become a doctor, if that's what you really want, and you're sure you have what it takes *inside.* For this reason, there's no sense talking here about the hypothetical effects of the *Bakke* decision, although we have all heard and thought about it. It is more important for you to know that there exists a whole network of senior professionals to help people like you. The questions that you cannot answer, they may be able to help you with. Just give yourself a chance.

My thoughts must seem very idealistic and naive to people who know how severe problems of racism, lack of money, and poor academic preparation can be. But I have known people who have done it, and they provide living proof that the will to succeed can conquer very many problems. But let me reiterate my earlier warning. No matter how motivated you are, *don't choose medicine as a vehicle for your social advancement, unless you genuinely want to be a doctor.* If you don't want to improve health care, take care of patients, or work in science, find another avenue for your energy. You have to be dedicated. There's no way around it. Now get going and good luck.

I have always had trouble dealing with concepts of "minority" and "majority." Maybe it goes back to my old math block. But I do know that there are a large number of "blue-collar kids" out there who feel as if *they* are a minority, a *poor* minority. Everything dealt with in this chapter applies to you, too. The basic truth is: Everyone is needed. Medicine does not have to be a private patrimony willed to elder sons by influential daddies. It can be your profession, too—and your patients'.

Now here are some thoughts and observations for those of you who have already identified with the gay community, either because of your own sexual feelings or your empathy toward classmates. Although we really don't know as much as we would like about the phenomenon of homosexuality, one thing is clear: Gay people have their own health needs, their own life-styles, their own risks and dangers, and their own feelings about how they want and need to be treated. Physicians who are not aware of this will "turn off" their unacknowledged gay patients and do them a great disservice. Although there are now educational movements in this country to make "straight" physicians more aware of their gay patients' needs and more sensitive to the way they deal with them, there currently exists a strong need for physicians with this special empathy to come forward. They are needed for direct patient care and to educate their colleagues.

If you need any proof of this, consider the experiences of one of our residents who worked several evenings a week as a volunteer in a large clinic in New York City that served gays in the greater metropolitan area. Noticing that he seemed to have an unusually faithful group of patients, he had a quick look at *all* the clinic records, like the good physician and detective that he was. Sure enough, the clinic had one of the lowest "no-show" rates ever recorded. (You should know that one vexing problem for most doctors and clinics is the large number of people who don't keep their appointments, or send advance notification that they will not show up. It really can mess up a schedule and cost everyone a lot of money.)

This physician wanted to know *why* his gay patients were so good about coming, particularly when many came from long distances, and suspected that it was because there were so few other places to which they could go without being put down or made to feel like idiots. After all, in other clinics gay women risked being put on birth-control pills by doctors who just naturally *assumed* that pregnancy was a risk for an attractive young woman! He is presently doing a study to prove or disprove his theory, and the results should be fascinating.

I do not know how admissions committees feel about gay medical-school applicants and couldn't care less. Neither should you, as it is nobody's business but yours. It is not cricket for them to ask about anyone's marital or parenting plans, and any questions in this area can be neatly sidestepped with the casualness they deserve. If you are gay and smart and have all the other attributes you know are necessary, consider yourself a needed contribution to the cause of keeping *all* Americans healthy.

Experience has taught us that physicians tragically injured or stricken by incapacitating illness can continue their medical careers by developing resources they never knew they had, switching to more compatible specialties, and/or limiting their work to the extent necessary. While few people would advocate persons with known severe handicaps *starting* a career in medicine, the proscription is not across the board. If you feel that you have what it takes to be a good doctor despite a known handicap, please seek guidance from appropriate individuals before you leave yourself out of the running. You might especially wish to interview some handicapped physicians. It takes one to know one.

Several years ago, I received a letter from a woman physician who was going to school in Mexico. She seemed like a sensitive and gutsy woman. Among other things she wrote:

> . . . I am the oldest of seven children and in my family women didn't go to college, let alone medical school. . . . I've been self-supporting since I was eighteen (I'm now thirty-one). I was ill-prepared for college, having gone to a commercial high school, but I was able to work my way through college (altogether nine years) and graduated from Queens College in New York with a B.A. in chemistry. . . . My four years in Monterrey have been difficult at times, but overall it has been a very significant experience for me. . . . I have almost always been the only American woman in my class. . . . Many of the American male students think I am a bit strange and don't miss many opportunities to make disparaging remarks. For the most part I try to respond in a low-key manner, because I learned long ago that when I try to reason with them it ends up hurting me more than changing them. . . . I will be beginning a Fifth Pathway Program (a year of supervised clinical clerkship required of returning American students) at Nassau County Medical Center in East Meadow, New York. . . .

She went on to discuss her interest in women's health, a paper that she was writing on the subject, and the fact that she needed help financing the rest of her graduate education. What she did not mention was something that I discovered quite incidentally several weeks ago when to my delight I noticed that she was featured on a television news magazine. Pictured on the tube, she came across as the lovely, warm, and delicious physician her letter had shown her to be. I also discovered that she was a victim of multiple sclerosis. Boy, would I like a woman like that to be *my* doctor!

Now I'd like to recommend a book you should not miss. Called *When Doctors are Patients*, it was edited by Max Pinner and Benjamin Miller, two Bronx physicians. Because the book is out of print, you may have to find it in secondhand bookstores, and it may even have to be "searched" for you. But it is well worth the bother, for it is a classic.

The book is a collection of essays written by twenty-two physicians, each of whom had to do battle with a serious illness, no two alike. It is fascinating to read how these men and women coped with severe illness, rising to great heights of heroism, and occasionally sinking to levels they would hate to see in their *own* patients. A number of them described how they had to retrain after learning that they would never see again, never hear again, would suffer progressive neurological damage, or would die within a few years. Virtually each one stated that being sick had made the business of doctoring a whole new experience for them, and had taught some much-needed humility.

It is for this reason that young people who have already learned this lesson should be encouraged to study medicine. It's too bad that so many people have to experience suffering to be truly understanding when treating it. But that is the way of the world. If you are handicapped, but strong and functioning well, consider medicine. Please. After all, we are *all* handicapped!

12.
For
Those Who
Love You . . .

Parents, sweethearts, and other intimates in a student's life can often make or break it. Nevertheless, students are rarely in a position to speak with authority on how they should be treated; pleas for understanding are invariably interpreted as self-serving excuses for the failure to meet expectations.

I had thought at first to give you some suggestions about how to deal with loving and necessary persons who have climbed up on your back and sit astride your neck with a horsehair whip in one hand and a cattle prod in the other. But it might be better if I spoke to them directly, while you do a quiet fade out. After all, if *you* say, "Don't bug me," you are just someone who's trying to get out of doing the dishes or fulfilling some other obligation. If it's said here, maybe people will listen with temporary respect.

If you wish to turn the next few pages over to the persons who will be needing them most, I'll be happy to be your advocate. You should read them, too, however, because the discussion may help you to see yourself as a member of a class with common problems, rather than one recalcitrant person who's just giving the folks a hard time. It was mentioned earlier that if you are to study medicine, you will have to frustrate, disappoint, and even hurt the people you love. They're entitled to react. It helps if both parties can sort out what they are dishing out and reacting to, and can talk it out together.

PARENTS FIRST

If medicine is being considered as a career for your son or daughter, the first rule, I think, is to keep your mouth shut. (Unless, of course, you're "talking it out together," and even then I'd do more listening than talking.) Nothing you can say will be right. Ambivalent young people will take anything you say, twist it around, and not scruple to hold it against you in later days if you don't behave now. Why give them ammunition? Age, experience, a cool head, a dispassionate attitude, an objective assessment of the realities, a mature point of view on the world, all mean nothing unless you are making a decision *for yourself*. Advice, by and large, is out.

"But," you wail, "how can such a young person be expected to make a decision like that without a word from me? I'm the parent, am I not? It's like choosing a marriage partner! His whole life could be ruined! She could be getting herself into a lot of trouble! This is not a career to be undertaken lightly!" Exactly. It is precisely *because* medicine is so alluring and so difficult, so exacting and so gratifying, that you must leave the bulk of the agonizing up to the object of its assaults and rewards.

The entire period of indecision, weighing of pros and cons, wavering back and forth, is best accomplished in fairly solitary fashion. Your student will have no help from parents once the grind begins, and if he or she cannot pass this first test of major decision making autonomously, you will have even *more* reason to worry about the future. Learning about medicine is like learning about sex—a certain amount of it has to come from the street.

It is important to remember that putting a gag on 90 percent of what you want to say does not necessarily render you a passive bystander to your loved one's decline and fall. You can provide a receptive climate for rational decision making. You can substitute *listening* for talking, the kind of informed, sensitive listening that will enable the student to hear his own words with *your* understanding. It is not *necessary* for you to talk. If you listen long enough, your student will hear everything you wanted to say. After all, if she's *your* kid, she's a chip off the old blockhead, isn't she? If he's *your* kid, he's basically a sensible person, isn't he? So, lay off!

The opening chapter of this book mentioned the possibility that some parents may be trying to relive their lives or seek fulfillment of their own unresolved fantasies through the lives of their children. This is a natural temptation, and if you suspect that it lurks in your unconscious mind, remember that there are greater crimes. Many feel that it is no crime at all to want your child to have a better life than you think you had. But the old adage holds true, *"Judge not your children, they were born in different times."* Moderately amended, it can be a reminder that what might have been good for you twenty years ago may not be good for your child now. Part of being a parent, I suppose, is accepting whatever happens with a certain amount of faith. In the last analysis, the decision will not be made by you or even your student, it will be made by time, college performance, medical-school acceptance, and the years that follow.

If your student is accepted in medical school, and you share his or her feeling that it will be a good career, you will have reason to be happy. But you will not yet be out of the woods. Consider, for example, the situation of a medical student living at home or within a twenty-mile radius of it. The parent may be forgiven for thinking that his or her child is more helpless and vulnerable now than at any point since nonambulatory infancy. It is well known that a medical student within reach of a maternal face can do a pretty heartrending imitation of a person in need of a warm shower, a good bed, some hot food, and probably some postprandial burping. Parents would have to be made of iron not to want to rush in with material support. After all, the very basic functions of life have to be reevaluated in light of a twenty-one-year-old adult who seems to have regressed so much under stress even self-feeding seems like too great a demand to fulfill.

Such parents fall into bad habits. They tiptoe around the house while "the Object" sleeps. They put a moratorium on the assignment of any household chores, errands, or duties. Risking their social reputations, they run interference with old friends, neighbors, and other assorted thieves of time. They become errand persons who take books back to the library, run the car in for a tune-up, and drop the cat off at the cleaners. After a while, they can hardly be blamed for feeling the way they used to during those old vacation days, longing for school to open in September so they could have some much-needed peace and privacy.

There are other reasons why they feel that their grown offspring have slipped back in time. The student is financially dependent, either upon parents or some remote government bank, at the same time that other young people are about to enter the work force and bring home a new set of wheels as proof that they are now mature citizens. The parents' ultimate financial responsibility enhances the tendency to continue to play the role of parent to a young child rather than a grown one.

Another important factor is that occasionally they will see their child suffer, a phenomenon as hard to bear now as it was when caused by the loss of a one-eyed teddy or a layer of skin right over the elbow. The suffering is caused by factors over which the parent can exercise no control—the fear of failure, the confrontation with meaningless death. Suffering in a child inspires the deepest parental feelings and can make people behave inappropriately in the consolation they offer and the solace they wish to provide.

I remember an example of this that occurred during my sophomore year in medical school. I was having some trouble with one of my subjects and was cursing softly about it on one of my visits home. Her brow furrowed in sympathy, my mother came up with the perfect solution: *"Why don't you let Daddy talk to the dean?"* I went through the whole horrified, oh-come-off-it-Mother! routine, failing to realize the source from which the inappropriate suggestion had come, or how reactive it had been to my very real pain. It was an excellent example of the anachronism of enforced "parenting" with a "child" of twenty-three!

It is important to realize that the seemingly increased need for parenting in the vulnerable medical student, coupled with the heightened need for independence during this period, is at the root of many, if not most, of the communications problems in families living together. Consider that medical students are frequently infantilized in their classrooms, because that is a prime pedagogical model of training in medicine. Even as they are expected to master enormous amounts of material relating to life and death, they are treated like high-school students. It is a schizophrenic existence, and one that really shouldn't be reinforced when they come home at night.

It is amazing that people in their twenties should still have to fight at work and home for recognition of their adulthood, but it happens all the time. A good parent of an adult human being who is functioning under stress will find a way to differentiate between proffering needed personal services and smothering the student with the unwanted restrictions of childhood. Somehow it should be possible to help and offer care without relating to the object of this service as one who cannot think independently, make personal judgments, and lead an autonomous life. Parents of medical students really should be given a badge, a guidance counselor, an orientation, and an organization of their very own. And I don't mean the PTA.

Let me point out something interesting to you. As I have been composing the past few pages, I find myself consistently stymied when searching for a word in the English language to refer to an adult child. There appears to be none. The "offspring" of a parent is referred to as that parent's "child," no matter how old. One can say, "my son," "my daughter," or "my child." But I can't find a noun to designate the *adult child*. Without a word to formally acknowledge the altered relationship as students reach their majority, we are justified in believing that the concept is rudimentary as well.

Grown persons who are still in school after the age of maturity, even the late age as defined by our culture, are vulnerable to a pe-culiar kind of imprisonment by those who love them the most—a benevolent, for-your-own-good kind of lockup. The luckiest are those whose parents can accept them as people who are now dif-ferentiated, for better or worse, and who must now stand or fall by what they are.

Although economic necessity will probably demand that more and more medical students seek training in a city where they can live at home and save money, this state of affairs can be hard on both parties. It is particularly true where four years away at col-lege have emancipated young people to a point of emotional no-return. Nevertheless, students who have elected other communi-ties are not exempt from the rule of eternal childhood. Although they are no longer within clutching distance, the space that echoes between them and their parents carries the vibes of what-ever went before. They can be haunted by what is not there, and given to fantasies more severe than realities imposed by parents living in the same household.

Here are some suggestions concerning the rights and responsi-bilities of parents of medical and pre-medical students. Since these will pertain for eight or more years, they should be well un-derstood and voluntarily assumed, for the desire to breach them will not be long in coming.

It would be helpful if parents could offer a love as uncondi-tional as they can muster, accepting as little as a low growl of rec-ognition for weeks on end as their only reward. If the grades of the "adult child" are inadequate to meet parents' exacting stand-ards, they will keep their mouths shut. If their "adult child" is a woman, they must not bug her about keeping up a social life, so that if she does flunk out, at least they'll have grandchildren. If standards of personal hygiene are faulty, they must refrain from poorly timed observations such as, "I don't care when that term paper is due, we are sick and tired of climbing over your garbage; either get your room cleaned up by 11:00 P.M. tonight or you can just move in with Joe Blow for the rest of the semester." If standards of conservation are not observed, they must withhold the temptation to unloose: "How many times do I have to tell you to turn the heat down and the lights out before you go to bed [at 3:30 A.M., but who's noticing]? Starting right now you are going to pay half the fuel and electric bills in this house!"

Parents have the obligation to refrain from using solicitude when it serves only to reinforce the student's self-pity and flight from independence. "You've studied enough, dear, now don't you think you ought to get to bed?" can be an absolutely lethal remark, if delivered at the wrong psychological moment. (At other times, of course, it can be as helpful as it was meant; knowing the difference is part of the art of adult-child parenting.)

Parents should help develop and honor a *taboo subjects list* that is invoked at all stressful times. This should include references to dieting, smoking, dating, periodic health checkups, choice of friends, choice of dates, spending habits, study time, inappropriateness or unacceptability of the student's emotional responses, politics, attitudes, and the like. In other words, the ideal parent should know when to step aside without going through life as if dancing on emotional eggshells.

Parents of students who are away at school should not use the telephone or the postal system as instruments of coercion. Acquisition or absence of periodic and frequent letters should not be interpreted as an index of love or rejection. The student should not be made to feel guilty on any one of a dozen counts through letters that begin, "Dear son or daughter as the case may be, I don't want to upset you and please don't let your mother know that I'm writing this, but I thought you should know . . ."

Parents should respect their student's need for privacy and not use financial support as a basis for nonfiduciary accountability. (Helping someone through medical school does not constitute a government program whose auditors are authorized by Congress to demand value given for monies received.)

Parents should learn to tolerate myriad paradoxical reactions in response to stress without feeling the need to point out the inconsistencies and self-defeating aspects of this kind of behavior. They should strongly sit on their temptation to relate how *they* would have handled a given situation, since they are only playing games with "the historical *if*." They should lead their own lives with a vengeance, if only in self-defense.

As already mentioned, parents of committed high-school students and early college undergraduates should temper their discouragement, leaving this unpleasant job to pros like me who have earned the right to debunk myths. They have every right to help their kids "reality test," but no right at all to impose any of their own feelings, however well intentioned. They are entitled to *feel* them, mind you. But they should padlock their tongues. It goes without saying that they should not "push."

In return for the scrupulous observance of these basic rules of courtesy, parents have a right to expect that their student will not play both sides of the fence. They may expect enough consistency and positive response to their sensitive handling of issues to make it all worth their while. This means that their student will not assume the "perks" of adulthood while demanding the spoils of childhood. It means that students will make a reasonable effort to understand the generation gap that properly should exist between consenting adults raised in two different eras, and will honor even that which makes utterly no sense to them simply because even parents have a right to their beliefs.

Parents have the right not to have a half-chewed-up experiment dropped in their oatmeal, when they have gone on record as getting sick at the sight of blood. They have a right not to sacrifice only to see the Object throwing his or her time away on unrelated nonsense. They're entitled to feel an ongoing sense of satisfaction and appreciation for what they are contributing to the cause.

Parents can help their medical students very much if they never forget how frequently they must deal with insecurity, worry, performance anxiety, shock, fatigue, and feelings of powerlessness. They should never fall for the myth of the glamorous, prestigious life of the student doctor. They should be sensitive to the many disguises students assume to cope with their intensive experience, and stand ready to help them take the greasepaint off when they need to.

SIGNIFICANT OTHERS

Everything I have said, so far, will hold equally true for sweethearts, spouses, and other close associates of either sex. In the latter case, the generation gap may close but dependency needs will still go demandingly on. A life that is running parallel and not twenty years ahead of the student needs its own kind of expression and nurturing.

In the old days, the wife of a medical student could accept rather readily the need for prostrating herself under the unyielding demands of the medical-education colossus. The steamroller of human expectation demanded it, and the theoretical rewards in the future made it all seem very worthwhile. It was generally accepted that for four, eight, or more years, the prime function of a medical wife would be to provide love, comfort, backup, financial support, and an unshakable ability to forego all personal needs and desires. The rewards were conditional gratitude, the heady thrill of unrelenting self-denial, and the approval of all civilized society. Of course, much of this has changed. Too many of those spouses ended up warped from years of stored-up resentment, atrophied growth potential, and isolation in a one-way momentum. Some of them weren't even spouses anymore.

If you are a woman who has fallen for someone who will be studying medicine, it's important to know why. Are you in love with the person, or the profession and the images it evokes in your mind? Are you interested in sharing the dream for perhaps the wrong reasons? Doctors are supposed to be men who spend their lives caring for others. There's a certain kind of woman who'd love to be married to such a guy. It's no picnic to discover that when he comes home at night, he's had it with giving everything to others and needs someone to take care of *him* for a change. Unless you have a touch of what those wives of twenty years ago had, you may end up with problem evenings. It's worth thinking about. There's no way you can beat being your own strong person, doctor's wife or no.

Take care of yourself first. Provide all the love and support you can, but only if you are also taking good care of yourself. It's important for the wife of a busy man to have interests of her own.

I think men who get serious about women in medicine are a special breed. It's true they may have some feelings about dependency, too. (Who doesn't?) But they certainly are not afraid to risk an unconventional marriage! If you are dating a woman who wants to be a doctor, and you decide to get serious, you'll definitely have to sacrifice more, fill in time with your own activities, and forego the experience of a relationship with a woman who makes everything secondary to the task of making you happy. Personally, I don't think you'll be missing much. We all have fantasies of being married to the perfect person who will satisfy our every wish, and we all know on some level that it can never be. Aren't you better off with a woman who cares about her world as well as her man? If you're in medicine yourself, you'll be getting a colleague and a lover in one "swell foop." Most of my friends from medical school are married to physicians they met during their training. They share memories and experiences given to few couples, and their marriages are among the most solid and enduring I have ever known. Perhaps it is my bias, but I think that men who have married women physicians are very sexy.

It does take some fancy footwork when two people with heavy career goals decide to split one address. I recently attended a conference on "The Two-Career Family," and how it adapts to enhance the mutual happiness and fulfillment of both parties. A knowledgeable speaker described the new, bivalent arrangement, in which both parties come home every evening, each prepared to take turns hustling the meals, exorcising the scutwork, and providing the emotional nurturing needed by the other. It sounded like a great arrangement, one in which a marital partner who'd had a bad day could count on coming home to TLC from a partner who knew the score. The idyll dissolved somewhat when a physician in the audience arose and asked plaintively, "Yes, but what do you do when you come home at night and you've *both* had a bad day." The roar of nervous and knowledgeable laughter indicated that the bugs in the Now Marriage still needed a good pesticide.

If you love a medical student or doctor, you will spend a lot of time dealing with these emotional issues. Treat them as serious business and nothing to be undertaken lightly. The best article I have ever read on the subject was written by two scholarly psychiatrists in Boston. Entitled "The Successful Professional Woman: On Being Married To One," it was published in the *American Journal of Psychiatry* in October 1977. With great humility and a rollicking sense of humor, they described what they had learned, and the comeuppances their male chauvinism had received during the course of their happy marriages to women physicians. Surely no greater love poem could ever have been dedicated to any woman! The kids didn't seem to be turning out so badly, either. If you have access to a medical librarian, try to dig that article out. It's worth it.

Perhaps it is unusual to write a book for young people considering a career in medicine and then include a whole chapter for their parents, friends, "significant others," even casual acquaintances. But medical students are so much helped or hindered by those who figure strongly in their lives, it seemed appropriate to involve you in what is, after all, a communal effort for the good of society. If I could think of any way to reach students' cats and dogs or other pets, I'd probably enlist them in the effort, too. Even goldfish.

Looking
Back
and
Looking
Forward

13.
Wrap-Up

Do you know that feeling you get when you've just walked out of an exam and all you can think of is the stuff you forgot to put down? And then you go home and your next of kin says (menacingly), "How do you think you did?" and you say (defensively), "I'm sure I haven't the slightest idea!"? You don't *mean* to snarl but you have been utterly outfoxed. You honestly can't tell if you've creamed it or bombed it! Well, I feel that way myself right now. I've finished my book, and all I can think of is what I forgot to put down. And whether or not I've creamed it or bombed it.

Nobody can go back and mop up an exam paper, but books offer more flexibility. So let me use this opportunity to introduce some offbeat ideas, wrap-up and expand on others previously presented, and assure myself that I've done everything in my power to clarify my message and deliver it to you.

This book has concerned itself almost exclusively with the twelve years of medical training because those are the years in which you will be expected to be a "student" for all or most of your working day. Those are the years in which your education will be planned, provided, monitored, regulated, evaluated, and ultimately utilized to determine your credentials to enter into the practice of medicine. It should be pointed out, however, that the close of the formal training period is not the end of medical learning, which continues until the day you retire or drop dead in your tracks like an old milk horse.

For generations, continuing education was a sacred trust of physicians. They were morally obligated to keep pace with new developments in science and technology because proper attention to patients demanded it. Nowadays, however, formal continuing medical education has become mandatory and codified for physicians, generally making ongoing courses and individual study prerequisite to license renewal or peer recognition. In fact, "C.M.E." has become big business in the medical industry. I get enough course and conference brochures in the mail each day (at hefty fees, by the way) to choke aforementioned horse. Skeptics point out that these are tax-deductible and often vacation-spot based, but they still represent time away from patient care for advanced (or remedial) study.

What all this means is that you're going to have to go on learning whether you like it or not. Therefore, you'd better *like* studying for its own sake. You'll never be able to stop doing it, no matter how many dues you may have paid during your twelve years. This observation is so elementary as to be almost ridiculous. But I'll take my chances and say again that if you really don't like to study, if you aren't naturally curious, if you prefer to memorize, and are basically too lazy to want to figure out complicated constructions, now's your last chance to get out and save face. Don't stand on ceremony. Run.

Now, I'd like to say something about nurses, without whom you will not last twenty-four hours as a clinical student, house officer, or physician. Nurses have a view of the medical profession given to no one else. For this reason, it is vital that you have some long discussion with experienced nurses, and not just the familiar people you know from your own physician's office. It's a bit like having a look at your girlfriend's mother to get an idea of what *she* is going to look like in twenty years. Unless you know what nurses think of physicians, and get their advice about how to educate and conduct yourself, you will always be operating in a sort of vacuum.

Nurses have become, in my opinion, the great tragedy of American medicine. Usually women who chose nursing for upward mobility, job security, or family tradition most sincerely loved to nurture, parent, and care for sick people. Accustomed to following the physician's prescriptions, and dedicated to improving their own nursing techniques rather than challenging from below, they received a rude shaking-up secondary to the development of the women's movement. Suddenly urged to express themselves, take charge, challenge physicians' errors, offer unasked-for advice based on superior bedside knowledge, they began to open up . . . only to find themselves facing the same rigid hierarchy and traditional superstructure so well-known to medical students.

Crushed between two immovable forces, nurses became subject to the most incredible amount of job-related stress. You can just imagine it! Understaffed, rarely thanked, brushed aside, not included in decision-making bodies, and with poor pay and long hours, their rage and frustration and inner distress grew. And they started leaving nursing in droves. Some went into administration, fostered by the new degree programs in nursing, and fixed their sights on more money and power. Some went into medicine. Some vainly sought private duty, temporary fill-ins, or other nontraditional assignments. And some, most, just went elsewhere. What a loss for all of us!

I feel guilty closing a book without giving you my opinion that you will be the inheritors of the crisis in nursing, and if you are not prepared to do something about it, you will find yourselves providing your own hands-on care for your patients (and a good experience it might be for you!), or seething in frustration as the wrong people botch up your patients.

Please talk to the nurses. Find out as much as you can about their profession and their problems, for they will be yours. Find out *their* perceptions of physicians. Develop some opinions about whether or not the physician is indeed "the captain of the ship," or if another model might not include the concept of real teamwork. Remember that you will be writing orders and walking away from your patients, while *they* will be watching the patient around the clock. In many ways, *they* are the healers most to be envied. And if patient care, in its elemental sense, has an appeal for you you may not have considered before, think about being a nurse instead of a doctor. I am completely serious. The image of nursing is changing, and I truly believe there is a place in this profession for people who thought they wanted to be doctors!

Before you leave the institution, try to talk to some social workers. They have important opinions about doctors, too. But don't believe *all* of it or you'll get depressed. They're a pretty jaded bunch! . . . And they're burning out, too.

Now, my wrap-up list reminds me to say a word about those whose job it is to help students when they run into problems, the advisers and caretakers provided by the educational institution for its family. These include student deans, student health physicians and staff, and faculty advisers. These people have an important role to play in offering guidance, support, information, advice, and validation.

Nevertheless, I advise you to be circumspect in your dealings with all of them. They all mean to help, but many are not in a position to do so, by virtue of the realities of their position. An institutional employee owes primary allegiance to those who offer security and paycheck. Many are, in fact, "double agents" who by definition cannot be of service to you without violating the interests of their employers, and vice versa. Without meaning to seem conspiratorial, I would simply advise you to watch what you tell people who may advertently or inadvertently use this information in ways you did not anticipate.

If you have a health problem, particularly a psychiatric emergency or upset, please do find a doctor or counselor on the outside, someone who will not be tempted to let your teachers or administration know of your trouble, someone whose files will be remote from those whose business you do not wish your problems to be. You will always find good people on site, but until you are sure they are appropriate people in whom to confide, take your burdens elsewhere. It's just good sense. You might want to read a case report on this subject entitled "The Psychiatrist as Double Agent," published a few years ago by the Hastings Center for Society, Ethics and the Life Sciences, in Hastings-on-Hudson, New York.

Students who have poured their energies into four years of premedical education can almost go crazy when they fail to gain admission to medical school. They'll be tempted to deny reality and make some desperate moves. Some will apply overseas and be accepted at a European university that has been turning out medical students for five or six hundred years. Of these, some will be able to transfer back after several years, or will find adequate post-graduate training to make them acceptable to the powers that be on licensing boards.

However, I want to call your attention to some new medical schools outside the continental United States whose academic base is very shaky, and whose main thrust appears to be tapping into the lucrative market of disappointed young would-be students whose parents can afford high fees. I think turning to these schools is basically a dumb move. So many have done it, there is now a growing lobby to have these schools monitored, recognized, and made legitimate. A number of factors, many political, will determine whether or not these schools will, in fact, be recognized by American licensing bodies. These include shifting trends in supply and demand, the growing power of parents' organizations, the expandability of American schools, and the vigilance of medical educators.

Please watch your step. You're treading on mercury when you go beyond the system, and your feelings about the rightness or wrongness of it will not affect the outcome of what happens to you. Medicine is hard enough without worries about whether or not you'll ever make it back to the States. Talk to Mexican, European, and Caribbean graduates . . . and the foreign-born and for-eign-trained physicians who have had a rather rough time of it in the United States.

Those of you who will be fortunate enough to be accepted to medical schools in the United States have been given a great deal to think and ponder about, if I have done my job and gotten a passing grade on this last test I have set myself. Only time will tell whether or not my worries about the impact of this book will have been well-founded. Although I have hinted at them before, let me share them with you.

My major concern is that I have presented a view of the medical education process that reflects its shortcomings too clearly and its successes too inadequately. Part of the problem is that short-comings tend to lend themselves to sharp critical analysis, and successes are too ephemeral to seize and describe with the warmth and enthusiasm they deserve. Most physicians, myself included, have had innumerable warm, deeply satisfying experiences in the exercise of our profession, and even in the acquiring of our educa-tion, but it seems maudlin and bathetic to try to describe them to others. Perhaps it is a remnant of that old ethic that forbids people to cry or express emotion or sentiment, when a few cold, descrip-tive words are traditionally more "manly." All I know is that some things wonderful are very hard to talk about. In addition, many of our best patient stories involve the role we ourselves played in comfort and cure, and few of us wish to appear as if we were blow-ing our own horns. Finally, many of the good things we remember involve our own therapeutic luck and cleverness, which we have trouble conveying to those who cannot appreciate the intricate detail of what we did to achieve our success and gratification, sim-ply because they have not had our training.

I do hope that I have been able to convey the satisfaction that comes from conquering difficulty. In the last analysis, this is the great reward of medicine, be it exercised in the care of patients or the completion of the training program that authorizes one to go out and do battle with their diseases.

A few months ago, I showed the first three chapters of this book to the husband of a colleague, who found them personally distressing. A poor Irish kid raised on the wrong side of town who became a professor of history, he confided that when he was young, he had desperately wanted to be a doctor. Only financial constraints kept him from his goal. (That's not going to happen to *you!*)

"These chapters make it sound like becoming a doctor is awful," he said in an accusatory voice, as if I'd sewn the flag on the bot-tom of my dungarees. "You'd better say something *good* about it or people who read it won't want to go to medical school!" Even after twenty years, the dream of what it was to study medicine re-mained untarnished in his mind, and he reacted as if to a personal assault on his fantasies! Although initially upset, I soon realized that I actually had accomplished my purpose—to make someone think seriously about what the educational experience entailed, even at the cost of sacrificing a few unrealistic fantasies. My friend's husband was clearly a distinguished professor of history, but it may well have been fortunate for him as well as the rest of us that reality got in the way of his pursuit of a career that proba-bly was not for him. I retained my chapters unchanged, and con-tinued to accept the risk that my presentation did not present a picture as whole as I could make it. If my book has been "skewed," it is up to you to fill in the missing pieces, from your own life and your own experience!

It is important to remember that our world offers many oppor-tunities to have a rich intellectual life, to be of great service to hu-manity, and to have fun while earning a living. Medicine is only one of them, and perhaps not the most important for the future we can anticipate. I have often wondered whether or not I would still choose medicine, if I were a student in the eighties. I have often identified careers that offer what medicine used to offer. For this reason, no one should have to feel that there is only one ca-reer choice of meaning for the future.

It is now six months since the summer rains came to New

Hampshire, and the pipes have long been frozen in the basement. But through these months I have been haunted by the remembrance of Anna and the role she played during that long night of nightmares. I have been thinking of her, and wondering which profession she chose. Did she marry, raise a family, then go back to school, as so many other bright women did? Would she have made a good doctor, after all, perhaps even a better one than some of her classmates who did make it through? Might she have been a good, alternate role model for some of the readers of this book? I keep wondering what message *she* would have had for you, if she could have been found and interviewed! For us, she is the great unknown, as are all the others who once wanted to be doctors but who went down another road in life.

No matter what your road, I wish you luck and blessings. If you become a doctor, be a good one. If you do not, remember this dream and keep it with you, for it will enhance whatever you do and become a part of your best self.

Suggested Reading

CHAPTER 2

Knight, James A., M.D. *Medical Student: Doctor in the Making.* New York: Appleton, Century, Crofts, 1973.

CHAPTER 3

Bluestone, Naomi, M.D. "Fire and Ice." *Medical Dimensions*, February 1977.

Osler, Sir William. *Aequanimitas and Other Essays.* Third Edition. Philadelphia: The Blakiston Co., 1947.

CHAPTER 5

Leikin, Alan. *How to Get Control of Your Time and Your Life.* New York: Peter H. Wyden, Inc., 1973.

CHAPTER 7

Balint, Michael, M.D. *The Doctor, His Patient and the Illness.* New York: International Universities Press, Inc., 1957.

Bluestone, Naomi, M.D. "The Melancholy of Anatomy." *Medical Dimensions*, October 1976.

Bluestone, Naomi, M.D. "Terror on the Training Ground." *Medical Dimensions*, February 1977.

Cassem, Ned, M.D. "Internship, Liberty, Death and Other Choices: How to Survive Life in a Hospital." *Harvard Medical Alumni Bulletin*, vol. 53, July/August 1979, pp. 46-48.

Cody, John, M.D. "The Arts versus Angus Duer." *The Role of the Humanities in Medical Education.* Monograph of the Society for

Health and Human Values (Symposium Proceedings held by the Bio-Ethics Program at Eastern Virginia Medical School). Philadelphia: SHHV, 1978.

Eichna, Ludwig W., M.D. "Medical School Education, 1975-79, A Student's Perspective." *The New England Journal of Medicine*, vol. 303, no. 13 (September 25, 1980), pp. 727-34.

CHAPTER 9

Bluestone, Naomi, M.D. Convocation address, Northwestern University Medical School, June 14, 1980.

Katz, Arnold M., M.D. "More on Pass/Fail: Letter to the Editor." *The New England Journal of Medicine*, vol. 303, no. 20 (November 13, 1980), p. 1182.

Lipp, Martin, M.D. *The Bitter Pill*. New York: Harper and Row, 1980.

Shem, Samuel. *The House of God*. New York: Dell, 1980.

CHAPTER 10

Bluestone, Naomi, M.D. "The Dating Game." *Medical Dimensions*, February 1978.

Bluestone, Naomi, M.D. "The Future Impact of Women Physicians on American Medicine." *The American Journal of Public Health*, vol. 68, no. 8 (August 1978), pp. 760-63.

Bluestone, Naomi, M.D. "Marriage and Medicine." *Journal of the American Medical Women's Association*, vol. 20, no. 11 (November 1965).

Bluestone, Naomi, M.D. "Miss Clairol Meets Her Match." *Medical Dimensions*, January 1978.

Bluestone, Naomi, M.D. "The Selling of Superwoman." *Medical Dimensions*, December 1977.

Walsh, Mary Roth, Ph.D. *Doctors Wanted: No Women Need Apply*. New Haven: Yale University Press, 1977.

CHAPTER 11

Miller, Benjamin, F., M.D., and Max Pinner, M.D., eds. *When Doctors are Patients*. New York: Norton Publishing Co., 1948.

Werner, Edwenna R., Ph.D., and Barbara M. Korsch, M.D. "The Vulnerability of the Medical Student: Posthumous Presentation of L.L. Stephens' Ideas." *Pediatrics,* vol. 57, no. 3 (March 1976), pp. 321-27.

CHAPTER 12

Nadelson, T., and L. Eisenberg. "The Successful Professional Woman: On Being Married to One." *American Journal of Psychiatry*, vol. 134, no. 10 (October 1977), pp. 1071-76.

CHAPTER 13

"Case Studies in Bio-Ethnics: The Psychiatrist as Double Agent." *The Hastings Center Report*, vol. 4, February 1974.

Naomi Bluestone

holds a bachelor's degree from the University of Delaware, a master's degree in public health from the University of Michigan, and a doctorate in medicine from the Medical College of Pennsylvania. Formerly Director of Community Medicine at the Bird Coler Memorial Hospital, and Assistant Commissioner for Chronic Disease at the City of New York Department of Health, she is Associate Clinical Professor of Community Health at the Albert Einstein College of Medicine. A consultant in medical communications, and a free-lance medical writer, Dr. Bluestone has recently undertaken a residency in psychiatry. She hopes it will help her to understand the second chapter in this book.